—— scale down

scale down

A Realistic Guide to Balancing Body, Soul, and Spirit

Danna Demetre, R.N.

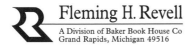

Fleming H. Revell
A Division of Baker Book House Co
Grand Rapids, Michigan 49516

© 2003 by Lifestyle Dimensions

Published by Fleming H. Revell
a division of Baker Publishing Group
P.O. Box 6287, Grand Rapids, MI 49516-6287

Fourth printing, February 2005

Printed in the United States of America

An earlier edition of this work was published in 2002 under the title *The Victorious Lifestyle* by Lifestyle Dimensions.

Library of Congress Cataloging-in-Publication Data is on file at the Library of Congress, Washington, D.C.

ISBN 0-8007-5878-1

Published in association with the literary agency of Alive Communications, Inc. 7680 Goddard Street, Suite 200, Colorado Springs, Colorado, 80920.

contents

5

—— acknowledgments

Any project, ministry, or significant accomplishment is always the result of people partnering together toward a common goal. A book is no different. It takes a team to get a message delivered with quality to you, the reader. And I surely must have the "dream team" of publishing. Thanks to my awesome agent, Chip MacGregor at ALIVE Communications, for his willingness to read a rookie's manuscript, take me under his wing, and find me the best publisher to deliver it directly to you. And what a team we have at Baker Books! My editor Jennifer Leep's enthusiasm and encouragement from our first meeting has been a wonderful blessing as I realized that the message of my heart was understood and enthusiastically embraced. Wow! Kristin Kornoelje made editing a breeze. Thanks to Cheryl Van Andel for her creativity in designing the book cover and for allowing a fifty-year-old the opportunity of a lifetime to actually be a "cover girl" of sorts. Thanks to John Sawyer for heading up a great sales and marketing team that goes the extra mile to get to know its authors and understand their message. There are so many others I have not met or acknowledged, whose hands have touched this book. Thank you.

Words cannot express the depth of love and appreciation I feel for my ministry partner and best friend, Terri Danley Podlenski. She has spent endless hours brainstorming, editing, proofreading, and encouraging me in every project I have undertaken in the past six years. In 1996 she started as my client in a lifestyle class, and we've been on an incredible journey ever since. Terri not only helped me refine and develop the teachings in this book, but she also has lived them victoriously since that first class.

I feel great appreciation toward my pastor and ministry partner, Dr. Tim Scott, for his commitment to teaching truth, his dedication to holding me accountable to the same, and his tireless hours spent reviewing my manuscript. The quality of the teaching in this book is directly influenced by the quality of his commitment to the Word of God.

I'd also like to express special thanks to Patti Milligan, M.S., R.D., for her contributions. Her twenty years of clinical and corporate nutrition experience lend high value to this book.

Let it be known that I not only have a publishing "dream team," I have a "dream" husband, Lew Boore. He never ceases to encourage and support me in all aspects of ministry. He sacrifices his time and convenience to allow me to express the message in my heart. For that, I thank you, my love. You are the BEST.

Most of all, I am thankful to our Lord and Savior, Jesus Christ, who is our ultimate reason to give thanks and praise. He is the author and finisher of our faith—the reason to live and breathe and exist.

—— introduction

— Dear Reader

My professional experience as both a registered nurse and fitness consultant has equipped me with a great base of knowledge to approach lifestyle change from a healthy and practical basis. However, the wisdom I have gained through my own personal struggles and God-given victory is the greater asset I have to offer.

If you purchased this book hoping to discover the truth about losing weight and realizing permanent lifestyle victory, you made an excellent choice. But before you begin to read or skim through the chapters, let me warn you. This is not a conventional weight-loss book. In order to achieve lasting change in both your body and habits, we're going to dig beneath the surface and address some important issues such as:

- understanding the balance of body, soul, and spirit
- realizing that you are what you think
- discovering the power of your true identity
- accessing the weapons to fight the "battle of the flesh"

I have written this book assuming you have a relationship with Jesus Christ. And while I believe that God's principles operate in the physical, mental, and spiritual realms despite our individual beliefs, your power source is yourself alone unless you know God through the redemption of his Son.

If by chance you don't know Christ, please go to the last chapter of this book, and I will be happy to introduce you. He promises to give you life . . . and give it beyond all you can ask or imagine. Not as the world gives but in a way that will satisfy you from deep within your soul.

While physical principles are essential to losing weight, most people aren't overweight because they don't know what to do. They are overweight because they don't know how to change. And there is no greater self-help book than the Bible to provide the truth we need for real change.

With that in mind, let's dig beneath the surface and begin our journey toward a victorious lifestyle. But let's start from the inside out. You'll see from my personal journey that I tried the "outside-in" approach first, with many failures and frustrations. I'll bet you have too. How about giving it a go God's way this time? It worked for me!

Praying for your victory,
Danna

P.S. By the way . . . before we get to the bottom line on how to decrease *your* bottom line, here are two weight-loss tips that always work: (1) Eat a little less and (2) burn a little more each day. And after you read chapter 1, take a quick spin around the block. It's the small stuff that adds up in a big way over time!

— 1
—— getting started
—

Hello and welcome to *Scale Down*! You've made the first positive step toward a lifetime of healthier living. I congratulate you!

— Starting Off with the Right Perspective

There are so many pressures to have a lean body in our society. At the same time, food and overeating seem to be a somewhat acceptable "addiction" in the Christian community. Where do we find a balance? We are called to present our bodies as "living sacrifices, holy and pleasing to God; this is our spiritual act of worship" (Rom. 12:1). Yet gaining an accurate biblical perspective and applying it to our lives can be very difficult.

Trying to change bad habits through sheer willpower and self-discipline usually doesn't work. In fact, it can be one of the most frustrating and overwhelming challenges we face. I know . . . I've been there. After years of struggling with compulsive, emotional eating and bulimia, I found victory and transformation by applying basic principles from God's Word and from the truth of how he designed our minds and bodies. It is a simple process, but quite honestly, it takes a little time and a daily surrender to God's power.

11

This is not a diet program. It is a spiritual journey that will equip you with tools, techniques, insights, and truth from God's Word. My objective is to help you make permanent changes in the areas of your identity in Christ, general health, fitness, and weight management. I am passionate about teaching truth in this book. And the truth is that we cannot change using our own power. But God is faithful, and his truth can transform our minds—and as a result, our behavior and body will follow. If you apply even some of the principles in this book, you will not only lose weight but also glorify God as you allow the fruit of his Spirit to become active in your life, in all of its dimensions.

— Basic Principles of the Program

Scale Down will equip you with principles and tools necessary to renew your body, soul, and spirit. But you must do your part to incorporate these positive changes in your life. A daily commitment to God coupled with persistent prayer is essential. You must be willing to participate actively until new behaviors become ingrained habits. As you begin, remember that you are not on a diet or a program that will end. You are beginning a new lifestyle that you will fine-tune and modify over your lifetime.

Give yourself permission to be human—don't expect perfection. And remember, every journey starts with a single step, and small steps taken consistently add up in a big way over time.

— The Body

Your body is your vehicle for life, so it's your responsibility to fuel up nutritionally for maximum energy and health. Your body also needs regular activity so it will run at optimal performance. While genetics and gender play a role in how your specific "machine" works, lifestyle is the greater variable. The daily habits

12

you maintain have the greatest influence on your health and weight management. The little things you do each day really *do* count.

In order to honor God with your body, it is important to adopt a lifestyle that makes sense, follows basic physical principles, and supports not only fat loss but, more importantly, good health. My program includes rational nutritional principles coupled with effective fat-burning strategies to help you maintain a reasonable body fat percentage. The two most important "bottom line" body principles we will focus on in *Scale Down* are:

1. *The bottom line in nutrition—in order to look and feel your best, your body needs premium fuel.* Don't try to micromanage your nutrition. Get the basics down first. Keep a reasonable and healthy perspective. Every improvement counts!

2. *The bottom line in fat management—calories in versus calories out.* You need to burn more calories than you eat if you want to lose fat. Most people need to decrease intake and increase output.

— The Soul

Our soul is made up of our mind (and intellect), emotions, personality, and will. The soul is driven by the mind, and all of our feelings and behaviors are a direct or indirect result of what we believe. It is our responsibility to use our intellect and the wisdom God gives us to identify the lies we believe and replace them with truth.

Whether we struggle with emotional eating, an inaccurate body image, or simply a lack of motivation, our best answers are found in God's Word. It is our responsibility to put truth into our minds and pray for the wisdom to apply it to our lives.

We can renew our minds by:

- taking our thoughts captive
- identifying the lies we believe
- meditating on truth every day

13

— The Spirit

We live in a fallen world and are, by nature, depraved sinners. But when we accept Christ as our Savior, his Spirit takes residence in our lives. We now have complete access to God and his power through Christ. Those who walk by the Spirit will not fulfill the desires of the flesh. However, this is not a onetime decision or event. His power is perfected in our weakness as we surrender each need to him. As we humble ourselves, he gives us grace for the moment.

In order to walk in the Spirit we must:

- learn the truth of our identity in Christ
- fill our minds with the truth of God's Word
- surrender our bodies, minds, and spirits to God
- humble ourselves and receive his grace and power for the moment
- pray for wisdom and the strength to apply it to our lives

— Lifestyle Success Strategies

As you read *Scale Down* and identify your weaknesses and stumbling blocks, don't try to implement each and every suggestion all at once. Pray for wisdom and choose one or two changes at a time.

Lifestyle change is not an all-or-nothing decision. It's an attitude and a series of small choices. So when life gets a little out of hand, simplify! In other words, focus on the most simple and effective techniques.

And when all else fails, just do something. Those little "somethings" will make a big difference in the long run.

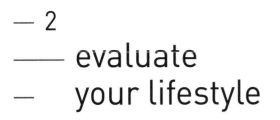

— 2
—— evaluate
— your lifestyle

You are about to embark on a journey. The following questions will help you understand your personal desires and level of commitment from the outset.

1. What do you hope to achieve with the help of this book?
2. Why is this important to you?
3. For whom do you want to make this change or improvement?
4. How will it change your life?
5. What will it cost you (in time, energy, money, etc.)?
6. Are you willing to pay that price?
7. Do you believe you can do this with God's help?

— Evaluate Your Lifestyle

Ignorance is not bliss! An ancient philosopher said, "Know thyself," and this isn't bad advice. After all, if you don't know what the problem is, it's hard to fix, and excuses and rationalizations undermine your achievement. Only the truth will set you free.

Begin by taking the following four self-evaluations, which will give you a good snapshot of your current strengths and weaknesses in four categories: (1) perspective/motivation; (2) fat management; (3) nutrition; and (4) fitness.

Spend about four to five minutes on each evaluation. Base your answers on your most consistent behavior or attitudes in the past three months.

- **Don't** rate yourself based on any changes you've made in the last four to six weeks.
- **Do** rate yourself based on your first impression.
- **Don't** go back and readjust your answers if you don't like the score.
- **Do** remember . . . this is a reality check. Just face the truth and move on.

Now it's time to face the music. Grab a pencil and be completely honest. No one has to see the results but you!

—— *Lifestyle Evaluation #1—Perspective/Motivation*

Based on the last three months, please rate yourself (0–Almost never; 1–Sometimes; 2–Often; 3–Always).

_1_ I see myself as a fully accepted and loved child of God.

_1_ My choices and actions are made based on my relationship to Christ.

_1_ I am thankful for the body God has given me.

_1_ I honor God with my lifestyle habits.

_2_ I take responsibility for my body's size, shape, and health.

16

___2___ My attitude is this: I am not my behavior. I am complete in Christ.

___1___ I surrender my weaknesses to God and rely on his strength for the moment.

___1___ My personal goals are realistic and honor God.

___1___ I take realistic steps toward my goals each day.

___2___ I know that with God's help, I can have a lean, healthy body.

___2___ I am aware of the lies I believe about my body, looks, and health.

___2___ I recognize and choose not to accept this negative thinking.

___1___ I renew my mind with God's truth each day.

___2___ I am a work in progress, and God delights in each good step I take.

___1___ Every day, I choose to submit my body, mind, and spirit to God.

___1___ I pray daily for God's strength and power to walk in the Spirit and not fulfill the desires of my flesh.

___23___ Add the total of all scores.

Scoring

40–48 Excellent! You have a godly perspective.

31–39 Good. Your perspective usually is working for you.

22–30 Fair. It's time to get a new focus . . . the truth!

< 21 Alert! Alert! Change your perspective now!

—— *Lifestyle Evaluation #2—Fat Management*

Based on the past three months, please rate yourself (0–Almost never; 1–Sometimes; 2–Often; 3–Always).

___1___ I feel in control of my food choices.

17

__1__ I measure my size by how I look and feel, not the scale.

__1__ I eat only when I'm hungry.

__2__ I stop eating when I'm full.

__1__ I understand why calories count.

__0__ I eat four to five small meals or snacks per day.

__0__ I limit my junk food, fast food, and desserts to less than 15 percent of my diet.

__0__ I am happy with my body weight.

__0__ I am happy with my size and shape.

__0__ I can enjoy "fun food" without feeling guilty.

__1__ I think about food only when I'm hungry.

__1__ I can see myself eating and living in control.

__0__ I walk or get purposeful exercise at least four times per week.

__0__ I am very aware of my choices and how they affect my body.

__1__ I say no to the latest diets or supplements promising quick results.

__0__ I know if I'm going to be lean, I have to take daily action.

__9__ Add the total of all scores.

Scoring

40–48 Excellent! You have a lean lifestyle.

31–39 Good. You're doing most things right!

22–30 Fair. It's time to take action.

< 21 Poor. Start with one step at a time.

—— *Lifestyle Evaluation #3—Nutrition*

Based on the last three months, please rate yourself (0–Almost never; 1–Sometimes; 2–Often; 3–Always).

_____ I think about what I eat and how it impacts my health.

_____ I have high energy to do all the things I want and need to do.

_____ I read labels and choose many foods based on that information.

_____ I eat two to three servings of fruit each day.

_____ I eat three to four servings of vegetables each day.

_____ I choose whole-grain products over more processed foods.

_____ I know how much fiber I'm eating daily.

_____ I drink ten to twelve glasses of water daily.

_____ I eat breakfast every day.

_____ I eat a good source of protein with my breakfast.

_____ I choose and eat lean protein with my lunch.

_____ I limit my empty calories to less than 15 percent of my total diet.

_____ I limit caffeine and other stimulants, such as over-the-counter diet aids, especially those containing ephedra and mau huang.

_____ I take a multivitamin supplement daily.

_____ I take an antioxidant supplement daily.

_____ I choose "healthy" fats in my diet, such as flaxseed oil, fish oils, olive oil, or canola oil.

_____ Add the total of all scores.

Scoring

40–48 Excellent! Your body loves you!

31–39 Good. You're on the right track.

22–30 Fair. It's time to try a little more high-octane fuel.

< 21 Poor. Your body is crying, "Help!"

19

—— *Lifestyle Evaluation #4—Fitness*

Based on the last three months, please rate yourself (0–Almost never; 1–Sometimes; 2–Often; 3–Always).

_____ I crave activity and find ways to move more each day.

_____ I enjoy exercise and how it makes my body feel.

_____ I have high energy to do all the things I want and need to do.

_____ I make exercise and activity a priority in my life.

_____ I understand the need for aerobic, strength, and flexibility training.

_____ I engage in aerobic activity four or more times per week.

_____ I take the stairs or park far away whenever I can.

_____ I monitor my heart rate and know I am exercising safely.

_____ I am injury free and able to engage in most activities.

_____ Being healthy and fit is important to me.

_____ I listen to my body and know what it needs.

_____ I wear appropriate and quality shoes for exercise.

_____ I have a very active life and am moving throughout the day.

_____ I work out my major muscle groups two to three times each week.

_____ I can easily touch my toes without bending my knees.

_____ I maintain strong abdominal muscles.

_____ Add the total of all scores.

Scoring
40–48 Excellent! You're a fit machine!
31–39 Good. Stay consistent.
22–30 Fair. Use it or lose it!
< 21 Poor. Take one small step and start moving!

Please note that the four personal lifestyle evaluations are repeated at the end of the corresponding chapters where the concepts are taught. I recommend that you retake these evaluations periodically in a different color pen to see the progress you are making.

— I've Evaluated My Lifestyle . . . Now What?

Now that you've evaluated your lifestyle and identified your most significant "speed bumps," it's time to take a look beneath the surface at all the dimensions of your life to determine why you are struggling. Some of the issues could be mental, physical, spiritual, or perhaps a combination of one or more. Your success depends upon your ability to understand key truths, make some important decisions, and implement consistent change. At the same time, you have to be realistic. It is impossible to work on everything at once. Prioritize your challenges and chip away at them a little at a time.

My job as your lifestyle coach is to give you some simple and realistic options. As a summary at the end of key chapters, I will give you "success menus" that will help you design a new lifestyle. As you make decisions about how you will eat and live, keep in mind that you can't build a brick house out of straw, nor can you build a healthy body out of sugar!

Don't get overwhelmed on your journey. Be patient and remember that small steps taken consistently add up in a big way over time. Your first small step is to start reading. Are you ready? Let's begin!

21

Part 1

—— Establishing Godly
Perspectives

— 3
—— the battle
— of the body

If you could change just one thing about yourself in the snap of a finger, what would that be? Has your outward appearance become an overwhelming burden? Do you feel like you are measuring the sum total of your self-worth by how you look? You are not alone.

Women of all shapes and sizes are agonizing over their bodies. Some of these women are clinically obese. Many are a little chubby. And quite a few simply are not meeting their own or society's expectations of the "perfect" body. But no matter where you fall in the spectrum, I have a message of hope and encouragement for you, one that will move you from a vicious cycle to a victorious lifestyle.

It's important to realize that change does not happen overnight. To effect permanent transformation, you must build on a solid foundation of truth. *Scale Down* is not a diet or a "program." It's a lifestyle perspective that will help you change from the inside out.

I've tried almost every diet that's existed. I've lost and gained the same twenty or thirty pounds many times. But about twenty years ago, I lost the fat and never gained it back. Most importantly, I was released from the bondage to my unhealthy attitudes and habits and was set free to experience life in a new and exciting way.

— I Hate My Body!

In frustration, I flopped down on my bed piled high with all the outfits I had tossed there over the past hour because they all "made me look fat." I buried my face in my hands and began to sob. I didn't want to go to the party anyway. I had *nothing* to wear. I felt fat, ugly, and defeated. And now because of my self-pity and emotional outburst, I felt superficial and immature as well.

I couldn't understand why a twenty-eight-year-old Christian woman could care so much about how I looked. I wasn't obese (although, if it weren't for my "problem," I would be). Regardless if I was a little chubby or incredibly obese, God loved me despite my outward appearance . . . didn't he? Then why did I have such a hard time liking myself? Why was I obsessed with my generous thighs, less than perfect hips, and advancing invasion of cellulite?

In defiance and despair, I retreated to the kitchen. I had a few hours before my husband would get home. I'd deal with my wardrobe issue and the party later. Right now I needed—or more accurately, demanded—chocolate. And so, like endless times before, I escaped into my vicious cycle of bingeing and purging. I had been a closet bulimic since I was seventeen. Nobody knew my secret. Nobody knew the extent of my internal battle, the daily struggle to get a handle on my eating, my thoughts, and my irrational body image. Nobody knew but me . . . and, oh yes . . . God.

At twenty-eight years old, I had been struggling for well over a decade. In reality, my bulimia had probably begun when I was only fourteen years old. That was the year I transformed from a thin adolescent to a more voluptuous young woman. All my friends were shorter and more petite than I was, and I found my five-foot, seven-inch height and 140-pound weight unacceptable and unattractive. I thought everyone noticed the "enormous" saddlebags I carried on the outside of my thighs. It was great living in Seattle in those years—swimsuit season was very short!

And so at fourteen years old, I began a long and frustrating journey that would lead me down many difficult roads, most of them dead-ends. In the process, I gained more weight as I hopped from diet to diet, believing each to be the perfect solution to correcting my imperfect size and shape.

I embraced many lies and discovered a few key truths along the way. The lies included the damaging notion that if I could get my eating under control and my body the right weight, I would be a totally fulfilled and happy person. I thought that no matter how I got the fat off, being thin would be sufficient motivation to keep it off.

After few successes and many failures over the next three years, I fell into the most devastating rotation diet of all time—diet pills and bulimia. After devouring enormous amounts of junk food, I would draw a line in the sand and vow never to binge and purge again. I became consumed with learning every tip to losing weight quickly. And the only way to make *that* happen was to get rid of my urge to eat. Those amazing little white pills really did the trick.

The next thing I knew, my boyfriend declared he would marry me since I was a lean 120 pounds. In my mind, I had finally achieved the perfect body. I determined to stay thin and was married four months later. Believe it or not, I actually took my bathroom scale on the honeymoon.

But even before we returned home, the diet pills seemed to turn on me. I became increasingly nervous and noticed frequent

27

heart palpitations. I knew the danger of amphetamines. I knew I had to stop taking the pills. So once again, I tried to use willpower and self-control to manage my weight. My new husband also did his part to help me. He pointed out every attractive, thin woman he noticed and reminded me, at every opportunity, of the things I didn't want to eat. He even turned down desserts on my behalf when we were invited to friends' homes for dinner. How *wonderful* to have such a supportive advocate.

Of course, he had no idea that the hidden problem I had was becoming an oppressive stronghold in my life. Since I felt so uncomfortable eating in front of him, I fell into my secret world of bulimia in order to "take control" of my conflicting urges to eat yet stay thin. When the numbers on the scale started to creep up and my clothes started to get tight, I reluctantly went back to the diet pills for help. I continued to lie to myself, saying, "I'll just get this excess weight off, and I'll never take these pills again."

By the time I was twenty-two and in my last year of nursing school, I had been through the cycle several times, yo-yoing between 120 and 150 pounds. But the last time I went back "once and for all" to diet pills to overcome a long bulimic phase and skyrocketing weight gain . . . was one time too many. I began to experience panic attacks. At first they were occasional, but soon they increased in both frequency and intensity. Within a year, I was living in overwhelming fear.

By the time I was twenty-three, the panic attacks forced me to realize that I could never take stimulants again. Gripping anxiety consumed my life. I thought I was dying. I thought I was going crazy. My fear of getting fat and losing my husband's acceptance paled in comparison to dealing with my fear of dying or losing my mind. It's a miracle I even made it through nursing school.

In my darkest hours of wrestling with my uncontrollable panic, I called out to God. And he answered. I learned the truth of Jeremiah 29:13, which says, "You will seek Me and find Me when you search for Me with all your heart." Understanding that Christ died for all my sins, my imperfection, my ugliness, my rebellion, and my self-sufficiency was an incredible relief. I had been so full of fear and shame for so long that I almost couldn't fathom the awesome depth of God's love for me. And while I had hoped that my new life in Christ would mean an immediate healing of my panic attacks, bulimia, and shaky self-image, God's plan was even better. Immediate transformation may satisfy our desire for comfort. But as it's been said many times before, God is much more interested in our character than in our comfort.

Although my initial desire as a young woman was to become lean and beautiful, God revealed many truths to me throughout my process of healing. The process took time, and, sadly, my first marriage ended before I could realize lasting victory. Yet God is faithful. He brought me to a place of celebration and acceptance of all he had given me in the physical dimension. He also helped me find victory over my habits and even discover a way to stay reasonably lean without becoming unreasonably obsessed with my looks. That is why I am writing this book and sharing my journey with you.

―― *What about You?*

What has brought you to the place you are today? What is going on beneath the surface in your life? When you were a little girl, how did you imagine your life would be as a grown woman? In those early dreams about the future . . .

- Where did you live?
- Who did you love?
- What did you look like?
- How did you feel?

And today . . . are those dreams fulfilled? What role has your body and self-image played in how you see yourself at this moment? As women, we are complex creations. Every one of us has a need for love, acceptance, security, and significance. Unfortunately, in our image-based society, our outward appearance is often the most common way we measure our value and worth. It's a lie, but many of us believe it!

Additionally, millions of women struggle with bondage to unhealthy habits—poor nutrition, lack of exercise, emotional eating, and bingeing. After years of dieting and going on and off exercise programs, many are frustrated and ready to give up, thinking that perhaps they *cannot* change. Many are continually asking:

- Am I thin enough?
- Am I pretty enough?
- Why is it so hard to change?
- What's wrong with me?
- Why do I feel this way?

I knew a young woman who struggled to find the right answers to those questions. Ultimately, she resorted to bariatric surgery to address her continued failure. But even that extreme measure did not produce the results she sought. Betty shared some of her deepest pain in the pages of her diary.

Tuesday, October 14, 1980. It's so disappointing when I come home and there's no letter from Steven. I haven't heard from him since July. He said that I sounded "fascinating." He'd feel differently if he'd actually seen me. What's the matter with me? Am I really that ugly and fat? I'm trying to lose weight. I don't think the operation was a complete success because sometimes I feel like I'm eating too much. I have to remember I didn't go through all that pain for nothing. If I can't lose weight after bypass surgery, I'm hopeless. I feel like such a loser.

Monday, November 3, 1980. *I want to be super slim for my brother's wedding. If I'm not, it's the real and true end for me. Life isn't worth living if no one will accept you. I keep remembering Steven and wishing he would just give me another chance—I don't want him to get married. I must be a real horror—when even my own brother won't fix me up. I don't blame him; he's probably ashamed of me. I just wish I had someone who liked me for me. I haven't thought of suicide for a while . . . but I'm so desperate to be loved. Well, diary, I've "bent your pages" long enough with my tales of woe. More tomorrow. Until then . . . I remain forever FAT!*

Wednesday, November 27, 1980. *I don't know what's the matter with me! My head is all mixed up. Here I was sticking to my high-protein diet for almost three weeks, then I blow it! Last night I went out with friends and I ate chips, popcorn, and ice cream. What is wrong with me? If I'm not thin by May, it's bye-bye Betty! I'm not a head case . . . but nobody understands. Why in this society is so much emphasis placed on your looks? Why can't guys accept you for your personality? I am so depressed. But I put up a good front! If people only knew what was going on in my mind. They would be shocked!*

Thursday, December 18, 1980. *I need someone so bad, but unless I lose weight . . . I'm hopeless. God, why don't you kill me? I'm not accepted in this world. What are you trying to prove by keeping me here? Are you testing my strength? Well, I am weak and worthless. I can't even name one worthwhile thing I've ever done. Help me! I am so desperate and disgusted with everything. I just want to fold up and die!*

Betty was my husband's sister. In October 1981, after spending six months partially paralyzed and on a respirator, she died

31

of complications from injuries sustained in a car accident caused by a drunken driver. She was only twenty years old.

Betty never found the answers. Even drastic surgical measures were not enough. That's because it is essential that we allow God to transform us from the inside out. It is important to do the right things with regard to nutrition and exercise, but knowing what to do is never enough. We have to change our thinking so new, healthier behaviors can become lasting habits.

—— *Is There Hope for Me?*

Despite the messages bombarding us from the world, we must help each other realize that we are so much more than physical bodies. There are too many Bettys who are living in despair. We must tell the truth and stop offering only physical remedies for fat bodies when there are so many struggling because they have starving souls.

Sometimes as Christians we believe that a simple profession of faith in Christ should cure us of all our problems. And when it doesn't, we think we are failures. I am amazed at the number of people who believe in their heads that God loves them but whose head knowledge has never traveled to their hearts. To know is one thing. To believe is another. We will spend a lot of time in this book digging into this very important truth, because what we believe ultimately influences all of our thoughts, feelings, and behavior.

While spiritual truth is paramount, we must also reject the diet industry hype. We must commit to learning the truth about how our bodies and minds work. Bringing all these truths into concert and moving them from simple knowledge to understanding and belief will have a powerful impact on our ability to make permanent changes in our lifestyle.

Thirty years ago it was easy enough for me to be lured into unhealthy fad diets and dangerous shortcuts. Today, more than ever, the multibillion-dollar diet industry is taking advantage of the fact that the battle of the bulge is an enduring epidemic. The

American public has allowed itself to be abused for far too long. After all these years, it is ridiculous how many people are still falling for the quick fixes and sudden-success advertising. This magic-bullet mentality continues to sidetrack many from taking responsibility for adopting permanent lifestyle solutions. Let me tell it to you bluntly—get over it. Magic bullets don't exist. Don't waste your time or money. Take responsibility. Unhealthy eating, inactivity, and excessive weight gain have created significant health risks for millions of men, women, and children.

— Your Body . . . Your Vehicle for Life

We must learn to use the tools God has given us to transform our lives—body, soul, and spirit. I love what Oswald Chambers wrote: "We are in danger of forgetting that we cannot do what God does, and that God will not do what we can do."[1] I think this truth applies to any area of life. In the physical dimension, God has given us an incredible body. That body is our vehicle for life. It is a tool to move us around during our time here on earth. It allows us to reach out and connect with other humans. And it will serve us only as well as we service it, much as we would our car. Think about it. This is the only body you will ever get. Unlike a car, you can't trade it in for a newer model. Until you receive your glorified body at Christ's return, this is it!

I sometimes wonder how God feels about how we care for our bodies. Perhaps it has some parallel to how my friend felt several years ago when she and her husband helped their daughter purchase her first car. The teenager was thrilled to have her own transportation. Despite the fact that the vehicle wasn't her dream car, it was almost new and in perfect condition. There wasn't a scratch, scrape, or nick anywhere. More importantly, it drove perfectly.

Within the first few months, she ran over a large piece of wood in the road and mangled her transmission. Then she accidentally bumped into a pole while trying to back up in a parking lot. The next thing her parents knew, she was parking the car all the way across the street. After a week, my friend got to thinking, *Hmmm, what's she hiding?* Curious, she walked over to check things out and found that the passenger side of the car had a huge dent in the door. Not long after, the brakes went out prematurely, the engine began sputtering, and the clutch burned out. One thing after another "happened" to that poor car. A year later, it looked like it was ready for the junk heap.

Imagine how those parents felt about the gift they had given their daughter. She had misused and abused it. Of course, they still loved her deeply. But she had disappointed them. Her care of her car demonstrated her lack of gratitude and sense of stewardship, so the last thing those parents were going to do was buy her a brand-new car. Instead, they helped her build some character through godly discipline.

I think God may feel the same way about how we treat (and see) our bodies. The body he gave you may not fit in with the "dream" body the world says you must have to be accepted and valued. It may not run like a fine-tuned sports car. But it is the only body you have. And if you see it through God's perspective and keep it fueled and tuned up, it will serve you well.

It took me way too long to stop looking for shortcuts. I learned there is a price to pay for a lean, healthy body. And it's paid in the small details of your daily lifestyle. Again, Oswald Chambers offered a pearl of wisdom when he wrote: "God will not give us good habits, He will not give us character, He will not make us walk aright. We have to do that for ourselves. Beware of the tendency of asking the way when you know it perfectly well."[2]

— All We Need to Live

God has provided all we need to reach our potential—whatever he has ordained that to be. He has given us food to eat, air to breathe, water to drink, and his Word to satiate our souls and spirits. If we think about the quality of his original resources, we realize they were perfect. Unfortunately, we humans have a tendency to pollute and destroy God's best. But if we simply go back to the basics in all areas—natural food, pure water, clean air, and the unadulterated Word of God—we will be amazed at what we can "grow"!

As we begin our journey, I encourage you to pray that the truths you read will make the difficult journey from your head to your heart. To realize any significant and godly change in your life, you must believe that God adores you and has answers to your deepest hopes and fears . . . even if you have failed again and again.

I'd like you to think of me as both a friend and lifestyle coach. I'm willing to be open and vulnerable in sharing the struggles of my journey, so I hope this will earn me the right to speak somewhat bluntly about your responsibilities for and attitudes toward your body and lifestyle.

Don't worry—I'll also teach you how to eat and move so you will burn that bothersome fat off your body. But a foundation of spiritual truth must precede any commitment to changing your behavior. I pray that you will feast on the principles from God's Word. Throughout these pages, I will share the truths I have learned that have changed my life from the inside out. I am confident they can change your life too. If you put him first and surrender to his power and truth, change will come, according to his perfect timing.

— 4
—— sweat
— the small stuff

In the next few chapters, I will be taking you on an exciting journey that I believe can transform your life. However, these initial truths won't directly address your primary reason for reading this book, which is a desire to change your body. So lest you worry that I will never get to the nuts and bolts of shedding those unwanted pounds, I want to share in this chapter some eye-opening facts about burning fat and changing your habits. Later, I will expand on each of these concepts in detail.

Despite the fact that I am giving you some of the basics up front, I think it is vital that you acknowledge one obvious fact: Most people have a decent idea of *what* to do in order to shed excess body fat. The problem is more complex—they don't know *how* to stay motivated to keep doing it.

My objective is to teach you how to lose weight permanently and healthfully. But I didn't invent these concepts. God created our bodies thousands of years ago, and they really haven't changed much since. They still respond to a set of physical principles God set in motion from the beginning. The truth is the truth, despite all the hype.

If you simply apply the principles you learn in these next few pages, you will be surprised at how effectively they work. I have an audiotape of a lecture I gave introducing these concepts to a group at my home church. Recently, I ran into a woman who had never met me, but by simply listening to the tape and applying the principles, she went from a size thirteen to a size five in less than a year, without dieting.

— Sweat the Small Stuff

Several years ago, a small book hit the market with a big impact. It was called *Don't Sweat the Small Stuff*. It gave great advice about letting go of things that really don't matter in the big scheme of things—especially the things that stress us out. But in the physical dimension, it's the small stuff that counts. You are not battling with too much weight simply because of the occasional binge, vacation, or holiday celebration. It's the little things you do every day that really matter.

Here's an interesting statistic. The average woman gains about twenty-five pounds between the ages of twenty and fifty. How many extra calories do you think she needs to eat for this to occur? You may be surprised. It's only about five calories! That's the equivalent of one breath mint a day. If you keep eating exactly what you're eating and only add that one mint per day for the next thirty years, you'll gain about twenty-five pounds. Sounds like really bad news, doesn't it? But the opposite is true as well. If you burn five calories more a day than you eat, you'll lose twenty-five pounds over thirty years.

But who wants to wait that long? Well, if we take the same principle and simply multiply it, we can accelerate the process. For example, if you burn one hundred calories more than you eat per day, you'll lose ten pounds in a year. Now let's work both sides of the "energy equation," both intake and output. If you eat one hundred calories less and burn one hundred calories more, you'll have a difference of two hundred calories each day. That's twenty pounds a year.

At first you may think your little lifestyle changes aren't making any difference because you don't see any indication on the scale. But it's happening. You just don't realize that those little lifestyle shifts really add up. People can move from a two-story house to a single level and gain ten pounds simply because they're not running up and down the stairs every day!

—— *Your Body—An Energy Bank*

The bottom line in losing excess weight is simply calories in versus calories out. I know that doesn't sound very sexy, but it's the truth. Your body is an energy bank. It stores and releases energy based on deposits and withdrawals. Most of us are making too many deposits and not enough withdrawals. This is just the opposite of what we are often doing in our financial lives. If we could reverse the two, we'd be on the right track—physically and financially!

Now you may be getting nervous. You're thinking, *Oh no, she's going to have us count calories!* Maybe yes, maybe no. That depends on you. I'll give you lots of options later for dealing with your energy account. For now, suffice it to say, calories *do* count.

I'd like to illustrate why understanding your calorie bank account is so important. Let's assume that I gave you a checkbook with $2,000 in it and sent you off to the mall. In this wonderful imaginary exercise, I'll give you two hours to spend it all. Wow, what fun! But I have a couple of important rules. You cannot subtract one single purchase until you are all done. And if you go over by even $1.00, you owe me $2,000. Most of us would fail miserably at this task. That's because we aren't good at accurately assessing what we are spending (or eating).

Have you ever gone to one of those large discount stores where everything is sold in bulk quantities? It's the kind of store you don't visit very often, so you usually make the most of each trip. When you finally hit the checkout stand, your cart is overflowing, and you know it's going to be an expensive purchase. However, you still aren't prepared for the grand total when it comes! The same is true as it relates to our body's calorie bank account.

The Bottom Line to Your Bottom Line

Our body is a perfect calorie-counting machine. It is absolutely accurate. When someone says, "I don't know what went wrong—I've gained twenty pounds over the last year!" I can tell you exactly what went wrong. The person ate more calories than she burned. A very small percent of the population has a metabolic challenge. And for those who do, it's rarely the whole issue. The bottom line is that the body counts every calorie. If you eat more than you burn, your body will store the excess calories as fat.

When people say they lost weight on this or that diet, the primary reason for the loss is always a calorie shift. Whether it's the Submarine Sandwich Diet, the Hollywood Diet, the Blood Type Diet, the Zone, the Atkins Diet, or the Ronald MacDonald Diet, weight is lost because you burn more calories than you eat.

Later I will explain in more detail some of the thinking behind a few of the more popular diets and why they don't make sense for long-term health and permanent weight loss. For now, please trust me; I am not alone in this concept of calories. The true professionals that understand human physiology agree—losing weight is ultimately about burning calories. After reading my chapter about burning fat to the max, you will better understand how your body likes to use its three sources of calories: protein, carbohydrates, and fat. And you will also understand why we need quality sources of all three for our incredible body machine to run and burn at top performance.

So how many calories did you burn today? The average American woman burns about 1,700 calories per day. At the turn of the century, she probably burned closer to 2,500 per day. That's a huge difference. Why? Her lifestyle was much more physically demanding. Our automated, sedentary lifestyles are dramatically different. Today, we need to simulate activity (move and exercise purposely to get that kind of calorie burn). Most people are not moving enough for good health, let alone burning all the calories they eat.

For almost a decade, I've used a little device called the Caltrac Activity Monitor that tells me how many calories I burn all day long.[1] Based on my age, height, weight, and sex, it calculates my resting metabolic rate (the number of calories I burn laying flat for 24 hours) and my moving calories (the number I burn in my daily activities). As a 50-year-old, 5'7", 140-pound woman, I burn about 1,400 calories laying flat for 24 hours. If I just go through my normal day without purposeful activity, I burn another 300 calories, for a total of about 1,700 calories. But you know what I found out? My appetite is about 2,000 calories per day. So if I eat 2,000 and only burn 1,700 calories, those extra 300 calories are being stored as fat on my body. Bummer.

Time to do a little math again. There are 3,500 calories in one pound of fat. So if you burn 500 calories more than you eat every day, you will lose one pound of fat each week. I recommend doing this as a combination of increasing output (calories burned) and decreasing intake (calories eaten). That's a lifestyle change. Try to find small ways to eat less and move more every day. You will be amazed at what happens over time. (By the way, I'll explain later why the scale is definitely *not* the way to measure this loss.)

My client Kathy is a great example of how to apply simple changes to realize profound change. In analyzing her lifestyle habits, she and I discovered 2 important issues. First, she was drinking at least 3 regular colas a day. That added up to about 350 calories per day. In addition, she rarely exercised. Over the

Establishing Godly Perspectives

course of 3 months, Kathy only had 2 to 3 colas per week and started walking about a mile and a half each day. She lost about 30 pounds and kept it off!

If you want to make a change that lasts, you need to find ways to modify your lifestyle, ways you can live with. There are many misconceptions about losing weight. The oldest is that you have to diet or make some drastic change to lose weight permanently. Think about your first diet. How old were you? What kind of diets have you tried? How many worked?

— The "Air Diet"—Hold Your Breath, Please . . .

Today, I want you to drop the word *diet* from your vocabulary. In fact, I think we should go on the last diet of our lives together, right now! I call it the "air diet," and it will help you recognize the futility of dieting.

It's only a forty-second diet, and all you have to do is stop breathing for those few seconds. Are you ready? Come on, just do it . . . hold your breath for forty seconds while you consider your thoughts and feelings by reading the following questions. Ready? One, two, three . . . go!

1. As your air diet begins, how does your body feel?
2. Scan your body from head to toe. Are you relaxed or tense?
3. How does your head feel?
4. How about your chest, shoulders, or back?
5. What are you most focused on right now?
6. How would you feel if I asked you to hold your breath for another thirty seconds?
7. Is your body getting more relaxed or tense?
8. Now what is the main focus of your attention?

Okay, that should be about forty seconds. If you haven't cheated already, go ahead and breathe. So, how'd you do? Did

42

you cheat? That's okay, most people cheat on food diets too. But if you really did the air diet, please answer these questions:

1. *What did you do just before you started the air diet?* I bet you binged! You took a big, deep breath of air. Why did you do that? You did it because you weren't going to breathe for a while. Think about your last food diet. What did you do the night before? (We never start diets at the end of the day. Have you noticed?) Most of us ate our favorite "forbidden foods." Why? Because we were never going to eat them again, right?

2. *How did you feel during the air diet?* Did you enjoy it? Most of us find holding our breath a little uncomfortable. We feel deprived and frustrated. We can't wait until it's over. Isn't that how a restrictive diet feels? Can you remember ever enjoying any of your diets?

3. *What did you think about most on your air diet?* Was taking your next breath on your mind? Apply this to diets. Doesn't it seem like we crave certain foods even more the minute we decide not to eat them? The best way to get yourself totally focused on a particular food is to take it out of your diet.

4. *As the air diet ended, what was the first thing you did?* You binged again! You took another deep breath. This time you had a physiological need for more oxygen. With some diets, you have a need for more calories, protein, or some other missing element. The binges on each end of the typical diet often do more damage than the benefit gained. We binge beforehand, then restrict our calories, and then binge again at the end, often gaining back the weight we lost. We end up in a vicious cycle. So what's the solution to all this madness? Stop dieting, of course.

Yet most of us are impatient. We want fast results. It may take years to gain the weight, but we think we can get it off in a matter of weeks. We give in to all the hype. So right now I'd like to explain why some of the most common weight-loss lies are so ridiculous.

— Common Weight-Loss Lies

—— Lie: *"You can lose weight fast."*

You didn't gain it fast, and you won't lose it fast either. In fact, you can eat 2,000 calories or more in an hour. Yet as I said before, the average woman only burns 1,700 in a day! You absolutely cannot lose a pound of fat per day. Yes, you can lose a pound on the scale, but who cares? That's water. If you starved yourself and ate nothing, it would take you about two days to burn off a pound of fat. (1,700 calories x 2 days = 3,400 calories, 100 calories shy of a pound of fat.) Throw away your scale. Get realistic. And make reasonable shifts in your caloric energy equation!

—— Lie: *"A supplement or drug will solve your weight problem."*

I wish it were so! We thought Fen-Phen was a wonderful thing. Now we know the truth. The risks were not worth the reward. Just ask the women who are concerned about their long-term health because they now have "waxy buildup" on their heart valves.

Have you ever listened to the list of side effects at the end of every pharmaceutical product advertised on television? Scary. So perhaps you'll just stick with the "natural" products such as ephedra, found in so many popular weight-loss formulas. Read the small print on those also. Just because they're natural doesn't mean they're safe or good for your body. Opium is natural. Cocaine is natural. Remember, I'm the one who got hooked on amphetamines to lose weight. Natural "speed" is not the answer. We simply do not need more stimulants in our bodies.

—— Lie: *"You can lose weight without exercise."*

You may hate the "E" word. Exercise from my perspective is simply simulated activity designed to make up for our outrageously sedentary lifestyles. If you are naturally active in your daily life, you may not need to exercise. But the point is that we all need to move purposely and with some intensity most days for the rest of our lives. If you don't get some form of aerobic activity and muscle work, your body will not burn fat efficiently. More importantly, you will not have the energy and endurance to enjoy life to its fullest.

—— *Truth: "Permanent weight loss requires a lifestyle change."*

Ask yourself this question whenever you're trying to get the fat off permanently: "Can I maintain this kind of behavior, activity, or type of eating most days for the rest of my life?" If you don't believe you can, then it probably won't work. Lose your fat the same way you're going to keep it off—through a permanent lifestyle change.

— The ABCs of Lifestyle Change

I hope the simple truths I shared about losing weight make sense to you. I can guarantee that the small changes you make will add up if you practice them consistently. And as you continue to read, you will discover more practical approaches to change in all the dimensions of your life.

Without the right attitude, belief, and consistency of action, nothing will happen. With that in mind, I want to address briefly the importance of your thoughts, or, more importantly, your beliefs, as you begin this new lifestyle journey. I will cover these concepts in more detail from a physical, psychological, and spiritual perspective in a later chapter.

To change your habits and behavior, you must first change your mind. I believe this is the most important principle for transforming our lives, and it is based on clear biblical teaching. In Proverbs it says, "As he thinks in his heart, so is he" (23:7

NKJV). The Bible gives us wonderful instruction and encouragement about what to put in our minds. If you keep hitting the same speed bump or brick wall—in your work, with your kids, with a habit, or whatever—you have to ask yourself what you really believe in that area of your life.

Perhaps you often say, "I can't remember names," and the truth is that you don't. Or you say, "I'm a chocoholic." If you believe you are, then you are. You believe you don't have control over chocolate. So again and again, that dominant thought takes precedence. That's why we have to be transformed by the renewing of our minds. We need to replace our lies and bad attitudes with truths that are first and foremost grounded in God's Word.

God's truth is incredibly powerful. But just identifying the truth is not enough. It takes time to replace the old lies. So ask yourself what are the lies you believe. Do you believe you can't be lean? What are your issues? Discover your lies and replace them with truth.

We're all different. As I've already mentioned, I became a compulsive, emotional overeater. I believed I was out of control with food, so I was. And, of course, in the whole bulimia cycle, every time I ate one more cookie than I thought I should, I figured I might as well eat the whole bag and throw up. It was powerfully destructive thinking. Over time I came to believe the lie that food had control over me.

What do you believe? Can you see yourself thin? If you've battled with your weight for years, you may not believe you ever can be thin. Lies sabotage us when we begin to believe them, so we must take control of what we allow to enter our brains. Some people get a little concerned that this might be some kind of New Age mumbo jumbo. It isn't. God has designed our brains to respond in specific ways to consistent messages. If these messages are negative or destructive, the results will be negative as well. Get in tune with all the negative messages and programs and tune them out. Get them out of your life. That's what victorious living is about—renewing your mind with truth.

Look to God's Word to validate your attitudes and beliefs. If your beliefs aren't in sync with his truth, replace them! It is also appropriate to create healthier messages specific to your personal issues or habits. For example, if you feel compulsive about eating every time you sit down to watch television, give yourself a new message: "When I sit down to watch television, I don't feel like eating." If you tell yourself that message long enough, you will start to change your thinking. This is a simple biological truth about how God designed your brain that I will explore in depth later. In the meantime, tune into your attitudes and internal messages. They may be leading you down a frustrating, even destructive, path.

— Get a New Attitude

In the area of lifestyle change, many of us need to throw out our past attitudes and embrace healthier perspectives. Popular pastor and author Chuck Swindoll describes the importance of the right attitude on all aspects of our lives:

> Words can never adequately convey the incredible impact of our attitude toward life. The longer I live the more convinced I become that life is 10 percent what happens to us and 90 percent how we respond to it.
>
> I believe the single most significant decision I can make on a day-to-day basis is my choice of attitude. It is more important than my past, my education, my bankroll, my successes or failures, fame or pain, what other people think of me or say about me, my circumstances, or my position. Attitude keeps me going or cripples my progress. It alone fuels my fire or assaults my hope. When my attitudes are right, there's no barrier too high, no valley too deep, no dream too extreme, no challenge too great for me.[2]

There are some common attitudes that sabotage your potential for lifestyle success. How many of these have you bought into?

—— *The "All or Nothing" Attitude*

This is the attitude that convinces you that Monday is the best day to start any new lifestyle change. And when the next Monday falls at the end of the month, you may as well wait until the first of the next month! All-or-nothing thinking leads you to believe that if you aren't "on" a program, you're "off." This attitude says nothing counts unless you're doing it all the way. Nothing is farther from the truth in regards to living a healthy lifestyle. Everything counts. And it's the small stuff day after day that makes the biggest difference.

Don't worry about tomorrow or even your next meal. Just live in the moment and surrender to God. When you blow it, move on. Don't give up and stay stuck. Receive God's forgiveness. (And please don't overspiritualize every bite you put in your mouth. That alone is making food much too important.)

Think of your lifestyle journey as a less-than-direct route toward your destination. Imagine you are walking across a room by taking three steps forward and then two steps back. This is what we do in our lives when we're trying to grow. Don't focus too much on the two steps back. Focus on the three steps forward and celebrate the fact that you *are* making progress! Throw out your all-or-nothing attitude and learn to adjust midcourse, cut your losses, and move on. And by the way, Wednesday afternoon after lunch is a great time to start your new lifestyle change!

—— *The "Quit before You Start" Attitude*

This attitude says, "I always blow it, I always end up quitting, so I won't even start this time." This destructive thinking grows out of years of failure. Don't become its pawn. Stop allowing yourself to wallow in past failure. Start celebrating every little success as a small deposit toward your future. If "quit before you start" has been your attitude for some time, I know the deep spiritual truths we'll explore in this book will be of great encouragement. Besides, you're reading this book, so you've already begun . . . why not continue?

The "Quick Fix" Attitude

Have you ever watched a toddler deal with delayed gratification? When they're hungry, they want food now! As adults, we understand that sometimes we have to wait to fulfill our desires. Yet in the area of weight loss, I am amazed at how people repeatedly pursue quick-fix solutions.

There is a prevalent attitude out there that demands a painless, fast, lasting, and no-effort solution to our fat-storage problems. People seem to think that if they can get the weight off fast, they will miraculously possess the inner strength, motivation, and know-how to keep it off. This is the biggest lie. The only things shrinking in America from this attitude are our wallets.

So the next time you're tempted to buy "Exercise in a Bottle" or "The Ultimate Fat Burner" . . . resist. Many of these products seem to give improvement simply because you believe they will. Scientists have consistently found that 30 to 40 percent of all patients given a placebo show improvement for a wide variety of symptoms. Placebos work if the person believes they should. This provides fascinating proof of how the mind and body work together.

The "It's Not My Fault" Attitude

"My husband is always bringing home Ben & Jerry's ice cream." "My wife won't let me put a gym in the garage." "The kids won't eat anything but hamburgers and fries." This attitude

49

blames everyone but the real culprits—you and me! Get rid of this attitude once and for all. Besides, all excuses are equal . . . and equally worthless.

Perhaps you have a thyroid problem. So do I. Take your medication and realize that your lifestyle is a much bigger influence on your weight than your slightly diminished thyroid function. Perhaps you come from a family of overweight people. So what? If you do the right things with consistency, you won't be like the others in your family. You may not be the leanest creature on the planet, but you won't be the fattest either! No one shoves food down your throat or forces you to live a sedentary lifestyle. Take responsibility and stop letting others influence your choices.

—— *The "I Don't Have Time" Attitude*

Talents and wealth may vary from person to person, but there is one great equalizer in life—time. While we are alive, we've all been given an equal allotment. We share the same sixty minutes of each hour and the same twenty-four hours of each day. The difference is in how we choose to invest our time. It's been said that we make room for that which we decide is most important. Choose to be the master of your time and find small, consistent ways to invest in your lifestyle. If you wait until tomorrow, it will never come.

—— *The Healthy Attitude*

Let's move on to a more positive perspective. A healthy attitude is one that finds a balance between current pleasure and future benefit. It allows freedom for flexibility and occasional indulgences without sacrificing health and wellness. A healthy attitude says, "It's my body and my choice. I'm choosing this."

If you need a little more motivation for making some positive changes in your eating and weight, here's a powerful fact that could dramatically extend your life.

50

In his book *The Hope of Living Long and Well,* Dr. Francisco Contreras states that eating a very nutritious diet of 30 percent fewer calories can add 30 percent more time to your life span, in addition to supercharging your overall health.[3] This means that if you expect to live to the average age of seventy-five years, you can increase that amount to approximately ninety-seven years just by eating less. In fact, he states that eating less is the only proven method to increase longevity.

I encourage you to forget about all the reasons you have failed in the past. Today is a new day and a fresh start. My purpose for this book is to help you find solutions, not excuses. It doesn't matter what challenges are holding you back. If you want to achieve victory, you must find solutions to those speed bumps.

— Discover Your Weaknesses and Design a New Lifestyle

Starting a new program without a good evaluation is like letting a dentist drill on your teeth before he takes X rays! As we explore the principles of healthy thinking, fat burning, nutrition, and fitness, you will have an opportunity to evaluate yourself at the end of each chapter to discover your weaknesses and begin formulating a plan of action in those four key areas (these evaluations also appeared in chapter 2). I encourage you to take the time to do the exercises. Without a plan, you are destined to fail. You don't have to take a lot of time. Just determine two or three things in each category that are the most important. Start there and add more when you are ready.

Here's a simple little method to visualize the positive changes in your lifestyle: Every time you complete a simple action, such as eating more veggies or exercising, put a penny in a clear jar. You will soon see the investment you are making in your lifestyle. (And if you really want to reward yourself, up the ante and buy yourself something special at the end of each month.)

In the next few chapters that follow, I will be digging beneath the surface to help you find the resources necessary to becoming transformed from the inside out. In the meantime, write down these lifestyle checkpoints and put them in a place where you will be reminded to review them every day.

- I am finding creative ways to eat fewer calories every day.
- I am finding simple ways to burn more calories every day.
- I am learning to eat for maximum energy and health.
- I am making purposeful activity or exercise a regular habit.
- I am identifying and changing my unhealthy beliefs and attitudes.
- I am building a foundation of truth from God's Word.
- I am becoming transformed by the renewing of my mind.
- I am learning to see myself and my goals through God's eyes.

I think we agree that there are no quick fixes or magic bullets. Instead, we must seek truth and take small steps to permanently change our bodies. It's not complicated, but it will take some time for those small steps to become our new lifestyles . . . something we can live with and even enjoy. Isn't that worth the investment?

— 5
—— balancing body,
— soul, and spirit

For this reason I say to you, do not be worried about your life, as to what you will eat or what you will drink; nor for your body, as to what you will put on. Is not life more than food, and the body more than clothing?

Matthew 6:25

— Finding Balance

Balance. It's a word most of us think we understand, but one that very few actually put into practice. I like this definition the best: a state of equilibrium. Is there symmetry and stability in all the dimensions of your life? I'm not talking about your home being in perfect order or all your to-do lists being completed. I am speaking of the delicate balance that generates an internal harmony between the body, soul, and spirit. You know when you have it. And you know when you don't.

The reason internal balance is so important is because each dimension of our lives impacts the others. If our bodies are out of balance, this influences how we think and feel. If our souls (including our minds and emotions) are out of whack, this generates unhealthy behavior. If our spiritual dimensions are neglected, we lose intimacy with God and are living only on our own steam. And as humans, that means we may have our priorities all wrong. The typical chaotic life of the new millennium, filled to the brim with urgency and activity, is a common symptom of a life out of balance.

When I spoke at a women's retreat on the subject of "Balancing the Dimensions of Your Life," I opened by asking them if they had made at least one of the following statements within the past week:

- Gee, I am so bored. I wish I could find something to do.
- Wow, life is so easy. I just don't have a care in the world.
- All my friends and family have it all together and totally energize my life!

Only one woman answered yes to the first question, and I told all the other ladies to give her something to do! Chances are you can't answer yes to all of them either. Do you ever feel like your life is a constant reaction to circumstances out of your control? That's the reality of life. So what are you going to do about it?

I have a confession. I'm a Type A woman, and I often live on the edge. I can pack my schedule so full of obligations and responsibilities that my hard drive (also known as my brain) begins dumping information randomly. I've found that there are pretty obvious signs and symptoms when a woman is living out of balance.

You know you're out of balance when . . .

Halfway through the day, you find your cereal box in the refrigerator and your milk in the cupboard.

54

Your idea of a relaxation break is laying back, kicking up your feet, and taking a forty-five-minute rest in the middle of the day . . . while getting your teeth cleaned.

You're ten minutes late dropping the kids off at school and twenty minutes late to work because you couldn't find your keys.

—— *The Overextended Life*

There are times in life when circumstances out of our control seem overwhelming. It is in these times that we learn to run to God and lean on him. We come to realize that so much of our lives are out of our control but that God has sovereignty over all things.

Yet much of the time our sense of stress and urgency is caused by our own doing. We simply give ourselves too much to do! And there is a price to pay. Edwin Louis Cole says, "The only true freedom we have in life is the freedom to choose. But once we choose, we become servants of our choice."[1] Sometimes it takes a lot of work and "undoing" to make up for a poor decision.

For example, I chose to enter the corporate world in the late eighties. Climbing the corporate ladder quickly, I was a marketing manager before I knew it, pushing toward a six-figure income. That income coupled with my husband's allowed us to purchase a larger home, better cars, and many other luxuries we had never owned before. But the enjoyment of those material "blessings" faded quickly as I realized that my rising income could not buy me what I really needed: time—time for myself, time for my family, and most importantly, time for God.

When I realized my perspective and priorities were off track, I wanted to make some immediate changes. I wished I could just quit my job and move on. But I had taken on financial obligations that my salary helped pay. So we had to go through the slow process of diminishing our debt and changing our lifestyle. Ultimately, we sold our home and moved to San Diego. I asked for a transfer, and with it, a self-imposed demotion so I could work from home. Two years later, I was able to quit my job and pursue my passion of writing and speaking full-time.

—— Hyper Speed . . . Hyper Stress

In this fast-paced world, most people's lives are moving too fast. We run out of time, money, and energy on a regular basis. Our relationships are strained, our minds overstimulated, and our bodies neglected. But the stressed-out, hyper-speed pace of the new millennium is *not* a requirement . . . it is a choice. And the price is very, very high. It can rob you of health, peace, and joy.

A life of balance requires sacrifice. We must invest in things that have long-term value over short-term gain. I've learned that we are a lot like airplanes—we can only hold so much luggage. If we get overloaded, we may go down. And despite our best efforts, when we take on too much, we don't really do well at anything. In essence, to live in balance, we have to minimize our load.

One day my friend Melody and I were discussing the challenges of time. We admitted that, like most people, we were in a constant juggling act trying to find enough time and energy for family, work, and ministry, not to mention a few moments here and there for things like exercise or relaxation.

It seemed like almost everyone we knew complained that there was never enough time to do all the things they wanted or needed to do. Full of wit and wisdom, Melody told me how she maintained perspective. "Danna, I just remind myself every day that there's a big difference between what I *can* do, what I *want* to do, and what I *need* to do."

"Yes," I replied. "And I just keep praying for the wisdom to know the difference and stay focused on what I need to do."

Melody gave me another dose of wisdom. "You know, when I start to feel overwhelmed, I go back to the basics and remember two verses. I fix my eyes on Christ (Heb. 12:2) and regard others as more important than myself (Phil. 2:3). Those two verses alone have such an impact on my thinking that I usually end up realizing so much of what I am busy about is often unimportant."

Melody had it right. Balancing the dimensions of our lives is first and foremost about an accurate perspective. It's about putting our relationship with Christ first and using wisdom from the Word to help us prioritize our lives.

—— *The "Martha" Complex*

Since I've already confessed to being a Type A personality, you can imagine how often I cringe at women's events when the speaker chooses to teach from the story about the "busy Martha." (No, I don't mean Martha Stewart, though she would be perfectly cast in the role.) I can just imagine the "original" Martha busily putting finishing touches on her handcrafted matzo ball holders as she huffed and puffed under her breath about lazy Mary sitting and chatting with Jesus.

I digress. I think the story more accurately goes like this:

A woman named Martha welcomed Him into her home. She had a sister called Mary, who was seated at the Lord's feet, listening to His word. But Martha was distracted with all her preparations; and she came up to Him and said, "Lord, do You not care that my sister has left me to do all the serving alone? Then tell her to help me." But the Lord answered and said to her, "Martha, Martha, you are worried and bothered about so many things; but only one thing is necessary, for Mary has chosen the good part, which shall not be taken away from her."

Luke 10:38–42

What did Mary understand that Martha missed? What are you missing? Are you prioritizing your schedule or scheduling your priorities? Are you putting off the essential in order to respond to the urgent? Are you often making comments like these?

- When I get caught up with my housework, then I'll have a quiet time.
- When the holidays are over, I'm going to get back to the gym.
- When the kids are back in school, I'm going to take that class I've been interested in.
- When I get some time, I'm really going to focus on my health, my friends, my life.

When never comes! I agree with the person who said, "We make time for that which is most important to us." Unfortunately, we often allow the loud, clanging demands of the moment to override the quiet nudging of real necessity. Those essentials do not become important to us until we are totally frustrated and over the edge. Or, sadly, when it is too late.

— What's "Balance" Got to Do with It?

What does this "balance" stuff have to do with losing weight or living a healthy lifestyle? Well, it has everything to do with it. Our out-of-control habits and unhealthy lifestyles are symptoms of lives out of balance. The problem is more likely our priorities and perspectives rather than our excess pounds.

If you are "balance challenged," chances are one or more dimensions of your life are suffering. And often that includes the physical dimension. You have good intentions about living a healthier life . . . *when* you get some time. Well, God allotted us all the same ration of hours each day—twenty-four. You'll never get more than that. Believe me, I've asked! So it's time to address the real issue—your perspective and your choices.

Juggling the Balls of Life

It's been said that life is like juggling many balls. Some of those balls (or life areas) are more fragile than others.

The Rubber Ball

Our work, daily chores, and to-do lists are much like rubber balls. No matter how many times we drop them, they just keep bouncing back. We may lose a job or two in our lifetimes. Our homes may not always be in "Martha Stewart" shape. Yet those areas of life just keep bouncing back to meet us. In these areas, it is difficult to cause damage that is irreparable.

The Glass Ball

There are other areas of life that are much more fragile and can be compared to glass balls. These areas include our physical, mental, and emotional dimensions, and our personal relationships. These "balls" can become scuffed, nicked, cracked, and sometimes even shattered if we neglect or mistreat them. In the physical dimension, our health may be permanently damaged due to poor nutrition, lack of exercise, and excessive stress. In our personal relationships, our neglect may result in broken friendships, rebellious children, or destroyed marriages. These areas of our lives need consistent care and attention. We cannot put off investing in them, because if they are neglected too long, they might break. The price is much higher, the risk much greater.

The Balloon

Our spiritual life can be compared to a balloon. We all have what has been called a "spiritual vacuum," a need to know our Creator. But before it is inflated, our spiritual dimension takes up very little space in our lives. Even as new believers, our spiritual balloon is underinflated. As we nourish our minds and spirits with God's Word, prayer, and fellowship, it expands and begins to take up a bigger part of our being. It influences our thoughts and behavior more and more.

A full spiritual balloon ensures that our perspectives about life are accurate by sifting all we think and do through an accurate biblical grid. As we fill our minds with God's truth, the Holy Spirit activates its power in our lives. As we pray about seeing ourselves and our lives through God's eyes, we begin to appreciate with fresh insight our identity in Christ. And as we seek to live within his will and choose to surrender to his power and plan, we find that many of our goals and aspirations lose their appeal. In other words, we begin to live out the Scripture that says, "Delight yourself in the LORD; and He will give you the desires of your heart" (Ps. 37:4). Our desires conform to his because we put our delight in him above our desires for self-gratification.

Yet without daily filling, our spiritual lives can fizzle out just like a balloon that is released without tying off the end. The spiritual dimension still exists, but it lacks vitality and influence over our body and soul.

—— *True Balance*

So how do we effectively balance the "balls" of life? Does living a life of balance mean we never drop any of those balls? Does it mean we live lives of consistent peace and order? Or does it perhaps mean we become ultraefficient superwomen with just the right time invested in each and every dimension? I don't think so.

It's been said we can be sure of only two things: death and taxes. In this life, you can be sure of two more: change and uncertainty. So the best way to balance a chaotic life is to keep your focus on the most important "ball"—the spiritual balloon. Fill your spiritual balloon through prayer, study, and meditation on God's Word, because only God's truth can provide you with an accurate life perspective. And despite how crazy and chaotic your life may become, you will have an anchor of hope that cannot fail. Even if everything is crumbling around you, you've "laid up treasures in heaven" that cannot be destroyed. The balanced life is not an easy, stressless life. It's a life that keeps bouncing back like one of those weighted punching-bag toys that won't stay down when you push it over. It's a life that celebrates the blessings that are already stored up in eternity.

——— Questions to Lighten the Load

Every day we are bombarded by dozens of choices. Many of them will be good things. Often in areas of ministry or family, we feel guilty for saying no to those good things. Yet we know that there are only so many hours in a day. How can we choose the best from all the good? Perhaps these questions will help you in that process:

- Will this help me know and love God more?
- Will this help me know and love my spouse more?
- Will this help me know and love my children more?
- Will this help me grow in loving others more?

Stephen Covey, author of the best-selling book *The Seven Habits of Highly Effective People,* made a statement that really made me think. He said something like this: "What one thing could you do (you're not doing now) that if you did on a regular basis, would make a tremendous positive difference in your life?"[2]

Think about that question: What one thing? The first thing that came to my mind was what Jesus said in Matthew 6:33: "But seek first His kingdom and His righteousness, and all these things will be added to you." If life is to have true meaning, purpose, and joy, we have to put first things first. As believers we know what that is. It is God, his Word, his plan, and his purpose. Yet too often we seek to fulfill our own desires and grati-

61

fication first. When will we learn? I challenge you to examine your spiritual balloon. Is it filled to the brim with air and expanding your mind and heart with truth? Or is it fizzled out and laying in the corner, lifeless, making very little impact on your life?

Have you ever had your car run out of gas or die while you were driving? Immediately the power steering is inoperable, and the car becomes very difficult to maneuver. You have to use a considerable amount of muscle strength to get it to move right or left. Living in our own power is like that. The "power steering" is not engaged, and we try to live effectively on our own strength rather than the Lord's. I once had an experience that went far beyond losing my power steering, and this frequently reminds me of the delicate balance of life. In reality, I have miniscule control over the bigger scheme of things.

My experience happened almost ten years ago, but it feels like yesterday . . .

— Steering Wheel Brings a Wake-up Call

Rushing out of the house, coffee cup and briefcase in hand, I was stretching the limits of efficient time management. I was off and running to a business meeting seventy minutes away—and I had sixty minutes to get there.

The freeway traffic was flowing fast for a Monday morning. As I returned my cellular phone to its cradle and placed my right hand back on the steering wheel, I felt an unusual heaviness falling into my hands. "Whaaaaaat . . . ? Oh, my Lord!" I said out loud.

The steering wheel had come completely off the column! My first thought was, *I'm going to get hurt today!*

I tried in vain to replace the steering wheel, but it seemed like time stood still. No control! Since I couldn't brake, I kept my foot on the gas to avoid being rear-ended by another driver.

My heart was pounding as I realized I had no options. My life and safety were no longer in my power, and my heart cried out to the Lord. "God, I can't do anything. It's up to you."

Miraculously, I cleared the first lane and then the second. I don't know where all the cars were for those split seconds, but they seemed to disappear. It was as if angels were guiding me across that treacherous route.

Still traveling at about fifty miles per hour, my car smoothly crossed onto the left shoulder, the front tire barely skimming the concrete safety curb. At that moment, I slammed on the brakes and came to a screeching halt, the barrier stabilizing my car and preventing me from spinning into the rush hour traffic.

Suddenly, I became aware of the loud whoosh of cars passing me at seventy miles per hour. Dropping the steering wheel into my lap, I raised my shaking hands and yelled, "Hey, everybody, slow down! Don't you know? You're really not in control of anything! You're not going anywhere unless God lets you!"

God captured my attention that morning. I was shaken by the possibility that it could have been my very last day on earth. Had I lived it to the fullest? Did my life really have purpose or meaning? Was I wasting too much time and energy on things that had little lasting value? I realized that day that I had been living out of control and without focus for far too long. And that day I made a lifetime commitment to live with balance and purpose. That meant putting first things first.

— The "One Thing" in Each Dimension

Once you've put first things first and are investing quality time with God and in his Word, it makes sense to consider the same "one thing" question in each dimension of your life. What one thing, if you did it well and did it every day, would make the biggest impact in each dimension? As you explore this question, don't make the answer too complicated. It's important to realize that you cannot implement every "one thing" in all areas of your life at once. In reality, that would make it "six things." Take a few moments to evaluate the six life dimensions and determine the "one thing" for each.

—— *Your Six Life Dimensions*

1. Physical
2. Material
3. Mental
4. Emotional
5. Relational
6. Spiritual

Was this insightful? Did any lightbulbs go off for you? The reason I'm asking you to ponder this question for each area is that one or two areas might be throwing your entire life out of balance. As you spend time with God, pray for the wisdom to know how to choose the most important "one thing" and invest time and energy in that area first.

—— *Putting the Physical Dimension in Its Place*

We have already established that the spiritual dimension is the most important. When that area is our greatest priority, we find that many things naturally move into balance. This is not to say we should neglect a direct investment in the other areas in the meantime.

> "Fitness of the soul should take priority over fitness of the body, but the two are not mutually exclusive."
>
> Bruce and Stan, *God Is in the Small Stuff*[3]

God must think a physical body is necessary and important because he gave you one for this time you spend on earth. It's important that we treat it well, so it will serve us well. It's also important to develop a healthy attitude about our bodies that honors God and conforms to his Word. I'm just so thankful we have a perfect, glorified body to look forward to in eternity!

Doing the simplest tasks becomes a huge burden when we are in poor physical condition. Remember the last time you had a headache, backache, or illness? Feeling miserable probably made it very difficult to do all you wanted to do with energy and enthusiasm. How we feel impacts our attitude and ability every single day. To live a full and effective life, we need to feel our best. So why is it we compromise the quality of our daily existence by taking such poor care of our bodies?

If we could see on a microscopic level what our habits are doing to each cell in our body and what the end result will be, we might just change. Or . . . we might not! Surprisingly, we are often more concerned about our immediate comfort and gratification than we are about long-term health and God's glorification. It's a sad commentary on our society when we lose our health to make money and then lose our money to regain our health.

To change our bodies, we must change our habits; and to change our habits, we must first change our thinking. (More about that in the next chapter.)

Your Body . . . A Living Sacrifice?

To realize lifestyle victory, you must have an accurate perspective about your body. If you are carrying around an unhealthy amount of excess fat, are eating poorly, or are never getting physical exercise, your perspective about your body may be inaccurate. The apostle Paul says in Romans 12:1, "Offer your bodies as living sacrifices, holy and pleasing to God—this is your spiritual act of worship" (NIV).

If you ponder that verse from Romans, you may be amazed to realize that presenting your body to God in a holy and pleasing way is an actual act of worship. Several times in his letters, Paul speaks about the body as a temple. Most often, he is encouraging believers to maintain sexual purity. And that is important. But I don't believe Scripture is exclusive to that one thing. It is a matter of stewardship. We honor God when we are grateful stewards of that which he has given. If you're like me, you've committed and recommitted your body to the Lord more than once in your lifetime. Perhaps more than once this very month! If all it took was commitment, we'd be perfect. That's why I've written this book. Presenting our bodies as living sacrifices is much more complex than a simple decision. However, a decision is an important starting point. Let's be painfully honest and take a blunt look at our bodies. What is the Bible really saying about our stewardship of this fleshly vehicle? Why not jot down a few thoughts below in the following areas:

The quality of my nutrition says: _____

The amount of food I eat says: _____

The way I move and exercise says: _____

The way I relax and sleep says: _____

The way I respond to stress or worry says: _____

In the Bible, God required all sacrifices to be perfect and without blemish. With respect to our bodies, I believe his view of perfection is far different from the world's. If you get a picture in your mind of the perfect, airbrushed bodies you see in so many magazines, you're not even close to God's image of a "holy and pleasing" sacrifice.

When a woman who has deeply desired a baby conceives and gives birth to a beautiful infant, she cares for that child as she would a precious, fragile gift. She nourishes it with food that will help him or her grow strong and healthy. She washes the child and soothes his or her skin with gentle lotion. She makes sure the infant gets rest and fresh air and is protected from harm. That is how we should treat our own bodies. We can honor God by taking care of our bodies as we would a beautiful baby. Not to the neglect of our soul and spirit, but in balance as a living sacrifice.

The Delicate Balance

As you see, there is a constant tension and influence that exists between body, soul, and spirit. Neglect of one will always impact the others. And while it is true that our earthly bodies will go away, they are important for living effective lives in this time. As we prepare to take a deeper look at the dimension of our souls, let's recap what we've discussed about balance.

Balance is not . . .

- an expertly managed lifestyle
- reaching all your goals
- success
- a stress-free life

Balance is . . .

- living with a godly perspective
- making choices based on truth
- practicing what we know is true
- leaving the results up to God

To build lasting habits, start with the spiritual and work outward!

Danna Demetre

Balancing the dimensions of our lives allows us to live with power and purpose as we put first things first. When we delight in the Lord and when our desires are in sync with him, we will be content with the results of our efforts. I hope you can appreciate why I believe this section of the book is so important to your potential of realizing lifestyle victory. Before we dig into physical truths, you must first fill your spiritual balloon to expand your soul for the journey.

----- *What Is a Victorious Life?*

A victorious life is one that honors and glorifies God. If you consider victory and success as being the same thing, you may be disappointed. But when you put first things first and seek his kingdom and righteousness, watch out . . . your goals may change. What is your ultimate objective? Do you want to please yourself and appeal to the world? Or do you want to bring God glory and live with great peace and joy in all the dimensions of your life? Do you trust him enough to surrender your goals and to pray that he will give you new goals that bring him glory? I am confident he will not disappoint you. But I admit that it's very scary territory. Let's continue the journey together.

— 6
—— discovering your
— true identity

Therefore if anyone is in Christ, he is a new creature; the old things have passed away; behold, new things have come.

2 Corinthians 5:17

— Who Are You?

So, who are you? What words best express the essence of who you really are? You may be a wife, a mom, a friend . . . the list goes on and on. And then there are all the things you do—your work, hobbies, and social activities. But does that really describe who you are?

Think about your life in all its dimensions. You have material belongings such as a house, a car, and other personal "stuff." You have a job or many responsibilities in managing your home. You have a family and friends. And more personally, you have a body that carries you everywhere and a mind that directs your thoughts and propels you to action. Is the real you hidden somewhere deep within that mass of gray matter?

— Stripped of Everything

Years ago, I read a compelling story of a man named Viktor Frankl.[1] He was a prominent Jewish psychiatrist who had endured the horrors of a Nazi death camp during World War II. Before the invasion of the Nazis, he was a wealthy, well-respected professional with a loving family, good health, and many personal joys. Then one day his life was stripped bare. Without warning, he was forced to leave everything he held dear and was thrown on a train crowded with trembling hostages chugging toward a dark future. That day, he lost all his material possessions, his career, his social life, and his family. I wonder, was Viktor Frankl the doctor the same man as Viktor Frankl the prisoner? Did the essence of his identity change because of his tragic losses?

These thoughts stimulated my already overactive imagination. With some Jewish heritage in my background, I imagined what it would be like if I had been a young girl living in Europe during those years. What meaning or identity would I cling to if I had been in Viktor's shoes? Would I have a sense of value and purpose when robbed of everything *I* held dear?

The truth is that I have never come close to that kind of experience. But someone I know has been through pretty tough times. It took some difficult trials to bring her to a deep and meaningful discovery of her true identity. While her circumstances were self-imposed, they were also a catalyst that produced profound results. As I visited her one rainy Saturday morning, her sweet, fresh-scrubbed face and passionate voice were distractions from the reality of her label—federal prisoner. Clearly, her eighteen months of incarceration had been well spent seeking eternal truths. She had new wisdom and a clearer perspective about life.

I almost laughed and cried when Jamie shared excitedly, "I never realized how little I need and what pleasure I can get from the smallest things. Today, I got totally jazzed about getting a brand-new pair of sweat socks and an extra blanket! And I was the girl that had to shop every time I had somewhere to go because I didn't feel good about myself unless I was wearing something brand-new."

What Jamie was beginning to realize is that the things she had and the way she looked did not define her. In prison, everyone is reduced to the same "class"—a jobless criminal. And everyone serves their time with the same social status—none. Whether the inmate is a wife, mother, career woman, or socialite, all their identities are left behind. All external relationships are cut off, with the exception of a few rationed minutes behind thick glass windows several times a month. Prisoners have one identity as they serve their time . . . a number.

Yet one thing this softened young woman had come to know deep within her soul was the truth of who she really is. She is so much more than a number, so much more than her possessions, roles, or relationships, so much more than her behavior, so much more than her sin. She is a child of God, deeply loved and completely forgiven.

She knows this to be true because she knows Jesus Christ as her personal Savior. "But as many as received Him, to them He gave the right to become children of God, even to those who believe in His name" (John 1:12). Despite her circumstance— the locked doors and uncertain future—she also knows that neither death nor life, neither angels nor demons, neither the present nor the future, nor any powers, neither height nor depth, nor anything else in all creation, will be able to separate her from the love of God that is in Christ Jesus our Lord (Rom. 8:38–39).

Would I have a sense of value and purpose when robbed of everything I held dear? I haven't been tested as Viktor Frankl or this twenty-five-year-old female inmate. But I've got to believe that if Jamie can grasp this truth from within a prison cell, I should be able to embrace the same truth with a strong and confident "Yes!" All I have to do is take God at his word. No matter what I lose, even my life, I am secure and have an eternal future. I am a loved and cherished child of God, and so is my beautiful daughter Jamie.

So let me ask it again: Who are you? The answer is essential to the quality of your life. If you simply know with your head that God loves you, that is not enough. You must believe with your very soul that this is true.

— What's Love Got to Do with It?

Love is an incredible motivator. Have you ever noticed how most brides lose weight before their wedding? It usually has nothing to do with dieting. Brides are consumed by something much more satisfying than food. They are consumed by love. They are motivated to do all they can to express their love to the man who has captured their heart.

> You shall love the Lord your God with all your heart, and with all your soul, and with all your mind.
>
> Matthew 22:37

When you fall deeply in love with someone, your mind is flooded with thoughts of that person. You reflect on your last moments together and wonder what he is doing and thinking right now. You anxiously anticipate your next meeting. You enjoy doing little things to make his life easier, without a thought about how it might inconvenience you. It seems in the early stages of love that many men and women can actually live out the words so beautifully penned by the apostle Paul in 1 Corinthians 13:4–7.

Love is patient, love is kind and is not jealous; love does not brag and is not arrogant, does not act unbecomingly; it does not seek its own, is not provoked, does not take into account a wrong suffered, does not rejoice in unrighteousness, but rejoices with the truth; bears all things, believes all things, hopes all things, endures all things.

Pure love is all those things. Pure love empowers us to do and be all God created us to be. It gives us a sense of significance, value, and purpose. It becomes the driving force and motivation behind all we desire. The love Paul speaks of is an agape love—a selfless pouring out of yourself for other people, not only your "soul mate."

Yet why does the intensity of love often stale, and our motivation to please those we care about wane? What has changed? Is it us or is it love? This is a complex question. And you may wonder what it has to do with balancing your spiritual dimension. Let me tell you, love has everything to do with it. Love is the essence of your spiritual dimension. If and when you fully understand the truths I am about to share, then you truly are on the way to experiencing incredible victory and joy in all dimensions of your life.

As humans, we naturally put ourselves in the center of our lives. Like little children, our natural default setting is programmed to focus first on me, me, me! Before we are saved, we walk in the flesh, because our spirits are dead to God. We may be kind and benevolent nonbelievers, but our motives and actions are man centered. Separated from God, we have no other choice. So when people disappoint us, betray us, or leave us, we move into self-protection, because the center of our universe is self. And too often that self-protection results in diminished expressions of true love as expressed in 1 Corinthians 13. In fact, without the Spirit of God living in us, we are incapable of real agape love. Our normal mode says, "You love me, I'll love you. You hurt me, I'll hurt you."

Unfortunately, we get a lot of emotional bumps and bruises in the journey to live our lives with Christ at its center. Too often in the process, we flop back onto our old perspectives, allowing our identities to become wrapped up in our roles and relationships. As young women, we measure our value by who loves us.

73

Later, we may invest much of our self-worth in our children, our work, or our ministries. But if you place all your need for love and significance in the hands of mere mortals, material possessions, or accomplishments, you will be disappointed. You may even be devastated or destroyed. I know. I did that once as a very young woman, and I lost myself for a season. But the next time I was betrayed, I stood on solid ground because I knew who I was in Christ.

— The Letter

I remember it was the spring of 1994. It was unusual for me to be home at 11:30 in the morning, even more unusual for the mailman to arrive so early. Life for me had just been unusual for the past few weeks.

I pondered my sense of emptiness and confusion as I strolled toward the mailbox. After years of running in the corporate rat race, I had finally taken an impulsive plunge into my own business. But from my husband's perspective, I appeared to be taking a suicidal jump into an empty swimming pool. Actually, Lew was quite angry and hurt that I had taken action without his blessing. Of course, it was something I'd been talking about for months, even years. I thought I'd told him how important it was to me. He thought he'd expressed the need to have a well-defined plan before leaving the perks and security of a management position.

He thought, she thought. Oh, well! Rationalization was a skill I had mastered during my "superwoman" years. *I* thought the time was right. *I* needed this change, and now was the time. *I* had negotiated a severance package. Why couldn't *he* emotionally support me in this? Was this why we were experiencing new struggles in our married life? For almost ten years I had felt loved and supported. I knew Lew was my best friend. We had always felt "connected." We laughed and called ourselves soul mates. But recently, I felt as if I was watching our relationship slowly disintegrate before my eyes.

Shortly after I had announced my resignation, Lew left on an extended business trip. He always traveled a lot, but this time he would be gone twelve days. Before his departure, I was caught up in a whirlwind of activities as I developed the marketing materials for my new endeavor. Videotaping and editing, brochures and business plans had filled my waking moments. I apologized profusely for overbooking my schedule and not being available to drive him to the airport. A quick hug and kiss and he was gone. Again I rationalized that those twelve days would be a great time to get all my work organized; then we could have some quality time.

Lew called me from his business trip, sounding oddly detached. He expressed an emptiness and concern for where our relationship was going. I responded with a mixture of surprise and anxiety. What was he saying? A week that should have passed quickly because of all my busyness became a string of endless days and sleepless nights. I became obsessed with the possibilities. Was it another woman, true discontentment, or was he simply falling out of love? My expressed fears and anxieties were placated with assurances of his love and commitment.

But a heaviness in my heart and spirit enveloped me as I reached the mailbox that day in 1994. As I emerged from my mental musings, I noticed that the mailman, who was driving up the hill and away from our community boxes, had left a pile of rubber-banded letters still sitting on top of our mailbox. *Hmmm, odd that he would drive off without them,* I thought. *These must be the letters that had been in the drop box for outgoing mail.* I figured they'd have to go out tomorrow since by now the mailman was long gone.

The bundled stack was too thick to stuff back into the narrow slot, so I removed the band and inserted the first letter. It was some type of magazine order with Lew's distinct and perfect printing. I inserted the second letter, and the third. Then my heart skipped a beat. The next letter looked like a greeting card in its soft lavender envelope. The precise printing again was easy to discern. It was Lew's. And it was addressed to a woman. By now my heart was pounding. I started to slip it into the outgoing mail slot. I really tried. But I just could not let go. Hurriedly, I crammed the other letters in and removed my personal mail from box number 12. The lavender menace stayed stuck to my left hand.

Safely inside my front door, I collapsed on the staircase. What was I thinking? What was I going to do with this letter? I stared at the writing, that printing I knew so well. Something was wrong . . . very, very wrong. I spoke to myself in a series of fragmented thoughts. "I have to know. I can't just go out and mail it. I must be crazy. It's probably a thank-you note to one of his business contacts. She's probably a grandmother! If I open it and it's nothing, I'll have to tell him what a crazy fool I am. If I open it and it's something . . ." That thought made me feel as if I had just tried to swallow a tennis ball.

"Let me be a crazy fool, Lord. Just let me be a fool." I ripped open the letter. It was one of those wispy, sophisticated cards with a message like "I Thought of You Today And . . ." My heart crumbled into a million pieces, and I hadn't read a single word yet. The note that followed explained a lot of things.

For weeks God had been protecting me from the lies and deceit. Despite an unusually strong gift of discernment, I had blindly accepted Lew's excuses and smoke screens. During that time of isolation, I had prayed that God would do surgery on my heart as I tried to figure out what was wrong with my marriage. I became convicted of my own complacency and personal ambitions. As Lew withdrew more and more, I began to hunger for the best friend and soul mate I'd once known. In his perfect timing, God profoundly delivered truth to me that spring day. His divine intervention exposed the truth that Lew so desperately needed to confess.

I gave God all the broken pieces that day, even though I wasn't sure how he would put them back together. Before I dialed Lew's pager number, I fell into a heap on the floor and prayed, "Lord, only you know the truth. Only you know how to put us back together again. You know the role I have played. You know how far Lew has crossed the line. What I know is that I love you and I love my husband. I also know I am capable of the same sin."

With his fullness of grace, God gave me a spirit of complete forgiveness. In that moment, his love poured out on me. I remembered the psalm that said God would not despise a broken spirit and a contrite heart (Ps. 51:17).

The ring of the phone jolted me into the present. Lew was returning my page. The "911" code had caught his immediate attention.

"Lew, I read a letter today. I shouldn't have opened your personal mail. I just had to. I love you. I forgive you. Please come home."

The slow journey back to restoration began with painful truth revealed. Then God's grace of hope and forgiveness fueled our human efforts. Recently, as Lew and I were walking along the beach holding hands, I shared how the Lord had helped me through those first painful months. And whenever I feel anxious about our marriage or the future, God reminds me of his purposeful intervention in our lives. I clearly picture the mailman driving up the hill, the bundle of letters sitting on top of the mailbox. And in the place of a painful letter, God delivers Jesus with his gift of forgiveness, peace, joy, and love.

—— *The Journey of Restoration*

Whether the holes in your heart are due to betrayal, neglect, or simply a poor concept of who you really are in Christ, you need restoration. We all do throughout this difficult journey called life. We need to know and believe the profound truth of God's love for all those who believe in the name of his Son. Without that truth penetrating us to the very core, we will seek significance and satisfaction in all the wrong places.

I know it must seem as if I have traveled far from the initial objective of making lifestyle changes that will transform your body. But I am much, much closer than you can even imagine. Remember, I am the woman who battled with emotional eating and bulimia for over sixteen years! There is only one way to come out of bondage to anything, and that is to step into pure truth, pure light, and pure love. The Bible says, "Perfect love casts out fear" (1 John 4:18). And, "Love covers a multitude of sins" (1 Peter 4:8).

—— *Choosing the Right Path*

The day I found out about Lew's affair was a testing time for me. Was I going to scream and yell and demand my rights or vengeance? Or was I going to seek the face of Jesus, follow his lead, and give what he had given me—forgiveness? My heart felt like it was crumbling inside my chest; my mind raced with all the imaginations of what Lew had done; but my spirit said, "Forgive."

Forgiveness isn't an exercise in self-righteousness. It is an act of obedience. I am no saint. I was angry; I was bitter; I was hurting. But I chose forgiveness. How could I do anything less when Jesus had forgiven me of every single sin I had ever committed?

At first when I cried or mistrusted Lew, he would angrily shout at me, "I thought you forgave me!" We both learned that forgiving and forgetting are two very different things. Trust and respect had been broken. It would take time to heal.

Initially, Lew tried to hide from his sin. He wanted to change churches, neglect friendships, and avoid talking about what had happened. Because of that, I learned an important lesson in those early months. I could not control anything about our situation except my own thoughts and actions. I had to do what God called me to do and trust him to convict Lew.

During the next year I experienced profound spiritual growth as I prayed and turned Lew and our relationship over to God. Prayer was the glue that held me together. Prayer was the power that connected me to the only control I had—trusting God. Slowly but surely he faithfully mended the broken pieces of my heart.

—— *Powerful Partnering*

Christian counseling was an important part of the journey back to wholeness. As Lew and I first entered our counselor's office, I was ready for her to help Lew change. Much to my surprise, she focused on me first! This very wise woman helped me see my role in making the marriage a true and lasting relationship. She helped me complete my journey to find my identity in Christ alone. That has not only made me stronger but more capable of giving and receiving love in a healthy way. That kind of wholeness helps me walk strong in every dimension of my life. I said "strong" . . . not "perfect." Like everyone, I'm still a work in progress. But, oh, the road is so much smoother when you know whose you are!

When we receive the free gift of salvation through faith in Christ, we are restored to fellowship as it was intended with our Creator. The perfect love of Christ's sacrifice washes over all our inadequacy, selfishness, and sin. We are forgiven for all time and eternity and judged righteous in the sight of God. Our salvation is secure. But our sanctification has only just begun!

As children of God, the Holy Spirit takes up residence in our being. We have all of the Spirit we will ever receive the moment we believe. Too many Christians believe that their sanctification is earned, much like a college degree. But it is when we fill our minds with God's Word, when we study, pray, and surrender our wills that the Spirit within us activates and motivates us to walk more consistently. That reprogramming allows us to fully appreciate our significance in Christ. Though others may let us down, nothing can separate us from the love of God.

— God Loves You

God loves you. Stop for a moment to really digest that simple statement. God loves you. Stop. Don't read on. Go back and pray that you can comprehend what that really means. We exist simply because our Creator chose to give us life. It is his love and desire for relationship with us that motivated him to bridge the gap between his perfection and our sin. It is his love that draws us to himself. The Bible says that we love because he first loved us.

—— *Run to the Truth*

When I am struggling with my own feelings of inadequacy or am feeling detached and alone, I find many areas of Scripture comforting. One of my favorites is Psalm 139. It grounds me in the truth of God's intimate and personal love for me.

> O LORD, you have searched me
>   and you know me.
> You know when I sit and when I rise;
>   you perceive my thoughts from afar.
> You discern my going out and my lying down;
>   you are familiar with all my ways.
> Before a word is on my tongue,
>   you know it completely, O LORD.
> You hem me in—behind and before;
>   you have laid your hand upon me.
> Such knowledge is too wonderful for me,
>   too lofty for me to attain.
>
> Psalm 139:1–6 NKJV

> For you created my inmost being;
> you knit me together in my mother's womb.
> I praise you because I am fearfully and wonderfully made;
> your works are wonderful,
> I know that full well.
> My frame was not hidden from you
> when I was made in the secret place.
> When I was woven together in the depths of the earth,
> your eyes saw my unformed body.
> All the days ordained for me
> were written in your book
> before one of them came to be.

Psalm 139:13–16 NKJV

I also find what J. I. Packer wrote in his book *Knowing God* both profound and biblically accurate. This is what he writes:

What matters supremely, therefore, is not, in the last analysis, the fact that I know God, but the larger fact which underlies it— the fact that *He knows me*. I am graven on the palms of His hands. I am never out of His mind. All my knowledge of Him depends on His sustained initiative in knowing me. I know Him, because He first knew me, and continues to know me; and there is no moment when His eye is off me, or His attention distracted from me, and no moment therefore when His care falters.

There is tremendous relief in knowing that His love to me is utterly realistic, based at every point on prior knowledge of the worst about me, so that no discovery now can disillusion Him about me, in the way I am so often disillusioned about myself, and quench His determination to bless me. There is, certainly, great cause for humility in the thought that He sees all the twisted things about me that my fellow men do not see (and am I glad!), and that He sees more corruption in me than that which I see in myself (which in all conscience, is enough). There is, however, equally great incentive to worship and love God in the thought that, for some unfathomable reason, He wants me as His friend, and desires to be my friend, and has given His Son to die for me in order to realize this purpose.[2]

Wow! Isn't that absolutely incredible? We are each created with an inherent need to be loved and know we have purpose. But most of us seek our relevance, our very identity, from our earthly roles and relationships. We seek intimacy and meaning more often from mere mortals than we do from a perfect God. By reversing our priorities, we make ourselves vulnerable to heartbreak and disappointment. People fail. Roles end. And then our sense of significance falters. But when a deep intimacy with God is our first priority, we have a foundation that can never be shaken. Even when the rug of life is pulled out from under us, we have a solid rock that keeps us strong—the unconditional love and acceptance of a perfect Father.

You Are Not Your Behavior

At the moment of your spiritual rebirth, you become totally identified with Christ. You are no longer a sinner. You are a saint, a child of God. This fact does not refer to your behavior; it refers to your identity in Christ. You are no longer your own; you've been bought with a price. Now out of love and gratitude, you are called to offer yourself (including your body) as a living sacrifice, holy and pleasing to God. Why should you behave in a way that glorifies God? Because God is always right, and he knows what is best for you.

Nevertheless, your behavior will not always demonstrate the truth of who you really are. We will discuss this "battle of the flesh" in another chapter. For now, I want you to embrace one important concept. You remain a precious and pursued child of God even when you don't act like one!

When your child messes up, does your love die? Do you disown him or her? Of course not! But a good parent does allow the consequences of poor choices to result in discipline that will move the child toward healthier behavior.

When my daughter Jamie was arrested for drug trafficking (for the second time), she called me from jail, crying and begging me to bail her out. It was one of the most difficult decisions of my life. She was close to hysterical when I said no. She told me she hated me and would never speak to me again. It was a painful time. But I had to express my love in healthy ways. I prayed for her. I wrote to her. And finally, despite her threats to refuse me, I visited her. Today, eighteen months later, our relationship is strong. She knows how deeply I love her. I know she loves me.

I loved Jamie despite her behavior, and I always will, even if she falls to the depths again. I choose Jamie. She is a gift from God. I choose to love her. And God chooses to love you, no matter what.

— I Choose You

One day while I was exercising (more about my TV exercise later), I watched a "reality" television show called *The Bachelor.* I was intrigued by its premise. An attractive young bachelor was presented with the challenge to find the "perfect wife" from among twenty or more women who had been selected based on criteria he'd provided. Over the course of many episodes, he would eliminate candidates until he had chosen only one that potentially would become his wife.

As the show progressed, he reduced his choice to his top five candidates. At the end of each episode, he would present a single red rose to those he wanted to pursue and "reject" just one. I was uncomfortable watching the women's faces as they waited for his decision. There was something in me that wanted to scream, "This isn't fair! He's got all this power and nothing to lose." Why would these women subject themselves to this kind of potential rejection? Sure, he was an apparently nice and definitely handsome young man. But choosing an intimate relationship this way . . . it just wasn't right! Was it?

In the end, he struggled with his decision and seemed genuinely concerned about finding the "right one." A lonely and rejected young lady rode off alone in the limousine just as the others had before her, while he embraced his chosen one, professing his adoration. One exhilarated chosen lady; many others rejected.

There isn't a way to build an intimate and deeply meaningful relationship and not risk rejection—that is, if the relationship is with another human. But if you're not experiencing a satisfying and intimate relationship with Christ, you have never really met him, or you have failed to spend adequate time with him.

If you know him yet don't feel loved and chosen, it's time you fully embraced the profound and limitless love he has to pour out on you. Every time you ask, every time you seek, he responds enthusiastically with "I choose you!" And he confirms his love, not with a single red rose, but with something far more precious, far more costly—his blood.

He alone can fill the gaps in our hearts left oozing with bitterness and fear from past rejections. But we must believe, and we must receive. If we were to marry the man of our dreams and never spend time with him or share our deepest thoughts with him, we would still feel alone. Draw close to God through Christ, and he will draw close to you. And while his love doesn't ensure that you will never be hurt by the "less than perfect" that roam this fallen world, it will sustain you and give you courage to risk your heart again.

If you've experienced rejection and betrayal, it's easy to project your bitter feelings onto another person. It's also natural to project those feelings onto God. Do not. He is incapable of rejecting you. Once you are his, he will pursue you with a passion. You may believe that you have gone too far, that you have to clean up your act before you have any connection with God. But that's a lie. While the sin in our lives does impact our fellowship with God, the key is to approach God in true repentance to restore complete intimacy.

As my pastor, Dr. Tim Scott, puts it,

There is a lie pervasive in our society that says that at some unclear, yet ever-present point . . . we've gone too far. We fear there is a line crossed, a sin committed, a wrong done that cannot be forgiven. There is no going home, no chance for restoration or reconciliation. So when is "enough, enough"? Is it three strikes you're out? Is there one or more unforgivable sins? If you've run away from God, I have great news for you. You've not gone too far. Whatever your sin, or series of sins, whatever lifestyle you've entrenched in . . . you've not gone too far. You can come home. That is not to say you should live with reckless abandon. There are consequences to poor choices . . . they can damage you and others. But it is never too late, you have never gone too far to reconcile with God. God forgives even though we grieve His Holy Spirit with our defiant and rebellious behavior. His love prevails even though there is a time of interrupted fellowship as His loving discipline guides us back home. Let us learn from Him, as we set healthy, yet loving boundaries for ourselves and others. It's never about you being worthy. No one is worthy. It's about the fact you are God's child. If you are out there on a limb and you feel there is no place to go and your heart is breaking . . . that you have gone too far . . you have not. You can always come home.[3]

God's grace is not permission to sin, however. Taking too much liberty with the concept of God's grace can lead to an unhealthy rationalization and attachment to sin that is destructive to our souls. We simply replace one lie ("I can't approach God because of my sin") with another ("My sin doesn't matter"). We must be diligent in studying and understanding God's nature and love accurately. Only then will we have full intimacy with the Father and a conscience that gives us power to live victoriously.

Realize Your Inheritance and Believe

It's difficult to live out our inheritance in Christ when we don't fully believe the truth of our transformation. Imagine that you'd been living in poverty for twenty years, not realizing that your

85

great-grandmother had deposited a million dollars in a trust fund for you seventy-five years ago. But once you realized this, what would you do with the truth? You'd probably act on it! It would be unbelievable if you never withdrew the money. But that's often how we live as Christians. We live as paupers instead of princesses. We live defeated instead of victorious. Why? We haven't embraced our inheritance. But how do we do that? Believe the truth! Simply knowing is not believing. When we truly believe, it transforms our minds and eventually our behavior.

The Spirit of God took residence in you when you believed, and he will bear witness and animate the truth of God's Word when you read, study, and meditate on it as if it were all you needed to sustain your life. Remember what Jesus said to Satan in the wilderness when Satan tempted him with bread? He said, "It is written, 'Man shall not live on bread alone, but on every word that proceeds out of the mouth of God'" (Matt. 4:4).

Spiritual, Life-Changing Victory Requires Daily Nourishment

To live a victorious life in all its dimensions, you must know who you are and become consumed with a passion to pursue God and his truth. The process of getting and keeping your "spiritual balloon" fully inflated is relatively simple. You need to nourish your spirit daily in five ways:

1. Pray as if it is the air you breathe.
2. Nourish your soul and spirit with God's Word daily.
3. Digest its truths through meditation.
4. Practice the presence of God.
5. Worship him in Spirit and in truth.

But there are so many distractions in life. It's so easy to believe the lie that we'll have more quality time to spend with the Lord and in the Word . . . later. Don't believe it. We make time for what's most important to us. I love what Christian psychiatrist William Backus says in his book *The Healing Power of the Christian Mind:*

A lifestyle that is too busy to pray speaks the truth louder than words. You don't really believe that learning to commune with God is good or you would value it more than you value your hectic schedule of activities.[4]

Tim Scott, my pastor, provided an excellent explanation of the process of how love motivates and truth transforms when he said:

"Love for God results in intimacy. And intimacy, combined with the truth from God's Word applied to our life, results in victory. Love is our motivator, and dependency on God is our power. Let your love for God and his for you become your primary motivator in all you do. This focus will ultimately transform your life as you build a strong and unshakeable identity in Christ."[5]

— 7
——— building a healthy
— body image

For man looks at the outward appearance, but the LORD looks at the heart.

1 Samuel 16:7

— Accepting Our Flaws

Do you like what you see when you look in the mirror? For me, it depends on what time of day I look! I certainly see a nicer reflection after a little makeup and hairstyling. Nevertheless, I don't think I've ever thought, "Now that's perfection. I finally look just right!"

The good news is that my appearance just isn't as important to me as it used to be. I've learned to maximize my assets and minimize my liabilities using a few wardrobe and makeup techniques I've learned over the years. And by God's grace, I've overcome my eating issues and maintained a reasonably lean body.

This has certainly helped me improve my overall body image. But most importantly, I am learning to celebrate with gratitude the body and appearance God chose to give me, despite the fact that this "earthly tent" is starting to give in to gravity.

Body image is a part of our total self-image. As we've already discussed, how we look seems to have more significance than who we are in today's culture. We are bombarded with magazine and television ads that say we need to look a certain way. For women, that image is an ultrathin model. For men, the pressure is much less, but it's there nonetheless. However, only about 10 percent of the population have bodies that even closely resemble the standard our society has placed on us.

Think about your early experiences as a teenager or young adult. What shaped your thoughts and feelings about your physical body? What messages have you been playing to yourself about your outward appearance? Women in our culture are under extreme pressure. Many men have higher expectations about their wife's or girlfriend's appearance than their own. Most men don't realize that the best way to help a woman reach her potential is to affirm her even when her body isn't perfect.

I had an interesting experience several years ago that illustrates this point perfectly. I was invited to be a guest on a local television station for a morning health segment. My topic was the truth about conquering cellulite. They put my number up on the screen, and I offered a free pamphlet for anyone who was interested. Over the next few days, hundreds of calls poured in. Later that week, I picked up the phone at our office and began a conversation with a fellow who had seen the segment. The conversation went something like this:

"Hi, I'm calling about that pamphlet you offered on the news earlier this week. I'd like to get one for my girlfriend," he began.

"Okay," I answered. "Did she ask you to get it for her?"

"Well, not exactly. It's just that, well . . . uh . . . I kind of think she could use it."

"Oh, I see," I replied.

"Well, will it work? I mean, do you really have ideas that can help her get rid of her lumpy thighs?" he asked excitedly.

"Sir, there is no magic cure for cellulite. The ideas in my pamphlet can definitely help reduce its appearance if they are implemented consistently. But many women are genetically predisposed to store fat in certain areas. Some very thin women can still have a fair amount of cellulite on the back of their thighs and buttocks. In general, women were designed to 'jiggle' a little. It sounds like this 'flaw' of your girlfriend's is really bothering you."

"Well, she would sure look better without it!"

"May I ask you a question?"

"Sure."

"Is there anything about your physical appearance that bothers you?" I asked.

"To tell you the truth, I am going a little bald. That bugs me a little."

"Great!" I replied enthusiastically. "I have the perfect solution!"

"You do?" he asked skeptically.

"Sure! This is what you do. Make a pact with your girlfriend. She'll never look at you from the eyebrows up . . . and you'll never walk behind her again."

Silence. Not the answer he was looking for.

> *Charm is deceitful and beauty is vain,*
> *But a woman who fears the LORD, she shall be praised.*
>
> Proverbs 31:30

But think about it. The disproportionate amount of time spent seeking the current "look" is really a matter of focus. And one of the best things we can do is change our focus. As they say, "Beauty is in the eye of the beholder." Will you behold society's image? It's difficult avoiding the constant bombardment of messages that influence how we perceive ourselves. However, it is essential if we are to celebrate with gratitude who we really are.

My good friend Diana Twadell has a very healthy perspective. Diana is an attractive, large-sized woman who writes for a women's ministry newsletter I publish. I think you will appreciate some excerpts from an article entitled "Beautiful People" that she wrote for our publication.

> As I stood in line at the grocery store the other day, I glanced at the magazine rack and there it was: *People* magazine's "50 Most Beautiful People" issue. I sighed and wondered what it would feel like to be on that list. And then I reminded myself that I have much more important things to do than sit around looking pretty. After all, I have a rewarding career, a Sunday morning class at my church, a budding public speaking ministry, and a host of other activities encouraging and mentoring women. I'm sure I'm much deeper than the "beautiful" women on that list.
>
> But I must confess that I tend to be a bit of a hypocrite when it comes to beauty. I may say that beauty lies on the inside and that appearance doesn't matter, but I tend to behave much differently. I downplay beauty and yet do everything I can to achieve it. I've noticed, though, that when these "beautiful people" are interviewed, they're not always content in their appearance. Most of us think they look great, but they think they could (and should) look better. The same seems to be true with success, wealth, knowledge and many other areas . . . the people who seem to have it all are always striving to obtain more.
>
> It makes me wonder: Can we truly be content in our own "beauty"? Is there such a thing as perfection? Most of us would agree that beauty is a subjective thing. . . . A visit to an art museum is a great way to observe the changing face of beauty. Some of the "beauties" on canvas would never make it on today's magazine covers. And some of today's super models would be considered too tall and skinny to sit for a portrait in the studio of, say, Rembrandt or Raphael. . . .
>
> Many of us feel . . . useless or worthless. . . . But what we see as worthless, God sees as priceless. And He longs to love us, heal us and encourage us to become the creation that we were originally designed to be.
>
> So, the next time I'm tempted to compare myself with the women on *People*'s list, I'll ask myself key questions about contentment, beauty and perfection. The answers lie in the principles God teaches us: putting ourselves in the hands of our Cre-

ator, trusting Him to know what's best for us, allowing Him to mold and shape our character and having faith that, in time, He can and will make masterpieces . . . out of us. The beauty that He achieves in us is not subject to culture or the opinions of others.[1]

— Seeing Ourselves from God's Perspective

Diana has described a grounded and spiritually balanced perspective regarding how we see our physical bodies. Clearly, building a healthy body image is most importantly about gaining an accurate perspective of who we are. That perspective is in our hands, or, more accurately, in our heads. I am not trying to discourage you from becoming your best lean, healthy self. But let's be honest . . . we won't all end up looking like Cindy Crawford or some Victoria's Secret model. It's an issue of genetics. Very few of us would struggle to stretch our bodies another four or five inches in height. It's virtually impossible (at least without platform shoes). So why do we try so hard to look like a body type that doesn't fit our own?

—— *You Are More than Just a Physical Body*

Did you ever try to motivate yourself to lose weight by putting pictures of thin women on your refrigerator? Or perhaps you even went one step farther and pasted *your* face on top of theirs. What an exercise in futility. To build a healthy and godly body image, we need to see ourselves from God's perspective, not the world's.

You must decide to invest time and energy in thinking differently. Look around you. How many of the people you see every day look perfect by today's standards? Not many. Just imagine if you didn't pick up one magazine, newspaper, or catalog in the next five years. What if you never watched one minute of television? What would your physical expectations be of your-

93

self? It would be much easier to accept and celebrate your body and appearance if you stopped comparing it to an unrealistic "standard."

As a young woman, I was terribly self-conscious about my thighs. I thought they were excessively fat and that everyone noticed my "saddlebags." I wanted nothing more than to acquire the long, lean, "Barbie doll" legs I had come to believe were the model of perfection.

I was oblivious to the reality of my naturally narrow waist and flat stomach. All I saw were my fat legs. Little did I know that all the girls who had thicker waists envied mine and never even noticed my "thunder thighs"! Ahh . . . the power of perspective.

Most women do not see themselves accurately. Like me, they become obsessed with what they view as their flaws. When our body image is warped, it's very difficult to let go of what you think you should look like and accept what God designed you to be. This is not to say that it is wrong to desire a leaner or more toned body. The key is to do the right things that promote reasonable fitness and leanness and accept the results with gratitude. To change your perspective, change your focus.

How Do You Really See Yourself?

Some of us cannot see ourselves realistically. No matter how much weight we lose, we still see a fat woman in the mirror. Despite the new outfits we buy or beauty tips we employ, we just never look good enough. This lack of contentment comes from deep-seated, unhealthy thinking. It took a lot of unhealthy messages to develop these destructive body images and it will take a lot more healthy ones to erase and replace them!

As with all areas of life, it is essential to do a reality check before you can move forward. What do you really think and, more importantly, believe about yourself? The following thought-provoking questions and exercises are designed to help you get in touch with your current body image. As always, we have to discover the lies before we can replace them with truth.

—— *Self-Discovery*

1. If you could snap your fingers and immediately change one aspect of your physical appearance in any way, what would you change?_____

_____

_____

2. Consider your total physical body in all areas and list three things that you like about your physical body. I don't mean just your physical appearance. Take a few seconds and force yourself to write down three things. _____

_____

_____

3. Was question #2 difficult to answer? If yes, why is that so? (You will discover some interesting things about yourself if you take some time to truthfully ponder these questions. Of course, there are no right or wrong answers. You're just doing a reality check on your current self-image.) _____

_____

_____

4. Consider all other aspects of yourself, other than the physical, and list three nonphysical things that you like about yourself. Perhaps you will focus on a talent or gift you have. Or maybe you're a great employee, mom, or friend. What first pops into your mind. _____

_____

_____

_____

5. Was question #4 difficult to answer? If yes, why? I have found that many people, especially women, find the first ques-

tion about their physical body harder to answer than this one. Why is it we are so hard on ourselves about our appearance?

_____

_____

6. Consider your total self, including your physical body, and list three things, and only three, that you do not like about yourself. _____

_____

_____

7. Was question #6 difficult to answer? For most of us, it is the easiest of all! It is not altogether unhealthy to have an objective, critical eye when we evaluate ourselves. However, most of us give ourselves far more negative feedback than positive. But we need to have a healthy perspective about both our strengths and weaknesses. Then we need to accept what we cannot change!

_____

_____

—— *Christ Confidence*

Do you believe God made you in his image? The goal of a grounded Christian is not a healthy self-image or empowering self-confidence but rather a deeply abiding Christ-confidence. And you gain that by learning to see yourself through your Creator's eyes. By taking an inventory of your current attitudes, you can identify your unhealthy thoughts and surrender them to God. Ask him to help you discard those falsehoods and embrace the truth of who you are in Christ—physically, emotionally, intellectually, and spiritually.

As you review the previous questions, think about your answers. Do they glorify God? Do your answers really reflect how you want to see yourself? Do they reflect how God sees you? If not, change them! Once again, the objective of this exercise is to help you identify any negative attitudes that may impair your ability to see yourself realistically as God sees you. We all have strengths and weaknesses. You have already learned that your ability to set healthy goals is dependent on what you believe about yourself. Change the negative messages by embracing the truth. First and foremost, refocus your attention on seeing yourself from God's viewpoint. He sees you as a complete person—body, soul, and spirit. He is most concerned about who you are inside. Yet he doesn't want you to disregard your body either. Pray that he will give you an accurate perspective and a grateful spirit.

Secondly, begin to rewrite your self-talk in this specific area. Start thinking and writing about yourself as if you already are the person God ultimately desires you to be.

— Self-Evaluation

The following questions will further assist you in learning how you currently view your body. Answer them as Never, Sometimes, Frequently, or Always.

1. I dislike my overall physical appearance.
2. I'm unhappy with the size and shape of my body.
3. I am unsure about my ability to make positive physical changes.
4. I am ashamed to be seen in a swimsuit.
5. I feel other people must think that my body is unattractive.
6. I compare myself to others to see if they are heavier than I am.
7. It is difficult to enjoy some activities because I am self-conscious about my physical appearance.
8. My discontentment with my size and shape preoccupies my thinking many times during the day.
9. I would feel okay about my body if _____ (a person's name) would accept me as I am.
10. My attitude and contentment is often influenced by how I look.

Results: Never _____ Sometimes _____ Frequently _____
Always _____

How many "Frequently" or "Always" answers did you have? Those are the statements you want to rewrite. Reverse the negatives to positive statements and tell yourself what you want to believe. For example:

"With God's help, I can change my body and accept myself."
"I celebrate who I am and realize my body is not the most important aspect."
"I see myself as a wonderful creation of God."
"I can enjoy life without always thinking about how I look."
"I am focusing on my strengths more than my perceived flaws."

Let's continue with our self-discovery by taking an imaginary journey. For this little "mind trip," I want you to throw on your most comfortable blue jeans, a jean shirt, and a pair of sneakers. Just get into your most comfortable clothes and relax. Everyone else on this imaginary journey is going to be dressed just like you! During this daydream, you will visit three different rooms, where you will meet three different types of women.

Room 1. The first room we will visit is filled with very talented women. They are all accomplished in the arts. They may be singers, dancers, artists, or accomplished athletes. And as you enter Room 1, you notice that they are all dressed exactly like you. Each person is smiling warmly and is excited to meet you. You have an opportunity to visit briefly with a few of these women. Perhaps your favorite recording artist or an author you've always admired is in the room. Go ahead, open the door and step inside. After a minute or so, ask yourself these questions:

Whom did you visit?
How did they respond to you?

Was the experience enjoyable or uncomfortable? Why?
Most importantly, how do you feel about yourself in the room?

Hey, wait a minute. Did you really go in there? If you didn't
. . . go back and check it out. I'll wait right here.
Okay. Now, let's visit the next room.
Room 2. In Room 2, the women are also dressed just as you
are, very casual and relaxed. This room is filled with highly intellectual ladies who are leaders in their fields. Imagine people
whom you admire and respect. Perhaps there is someone specific you have always wanted to meet. You have a unique opportunity to visit with one or more of these successful women.
Spend a few minutes in this room and then ask yourself the same
questions.

Whom did you visit?
How did they respond to you?
Was the experience enjoyable or uncomfortable? Why?
Most importantly, how do you feel about yourself in the room?

We have one more room to visit, so we'd better get going.
Room 3. Once again, the women are all dressed just like you.
As you enter the room, you notice it is filled with beautiful
women of all ages. Perhaps they look like Christie Brinkley or
Julia Roberts or Cindy Crawford. Just imagine all the women
that you think are beautiful. Now, back to our fantasy. (If you
happen to be a man, you are in a room with good-looking men
such as Mel Gibson or Brad Pitt. No jumping into the women's
room!) Now imagine yourself in the middle of this room surrounded by these gorgeous people. They are all incredibly
friendly and genuinely interested in chatting with you.

Whom did you visit?
How did they respond to you?

Was the experience enjoyable or uncomfortable? Why?
Most importantly, how do you feel about yourself in the room?

Before we leave, imagine for just a few moments what it would be like if all of a sudden you were all wearing swimsuits. Wait! Get back in there. Get in tune with your true thoughts and feelings. Ask yourself all the same questions. Okay, *now* it's time to leave. Let's get back to reality and address a few questions.

How did you feel in each of the rooms?
Did anyone in particular make you feel uncomfortable or self-conscious?
What was the most positive part of the imaginary journey?
What was the most negative?
What is the most significant thing you learned?

There is a very important truth I want to make sure you grasp. It is this: Despite your feelings or negative thoughts, you did not change as you entered each room and met the other women. You were the same person inside the room as you were before you entered. Only your perception of yourself changed. Often, we measure how we feel about ourselves by those around us— by their strengths and weaknesses or by their response to us. None of this is valid. You are a unique and valuable person with your own set of strengths and weaknesses. Some people are just a little closer to their potential!

— God's Perspective on Beauty and Our Body

It is easy to understand why beauty is so important to us. I'm sure we are all well aware of the endless images that reflect its significance. And research reveals that "beautiful people" get more attention. They are more likely to acquire better jobs, higher pay, and a host of other privileges "average people" don't receive. But you don't have to buy into the unreasonable emphasis on outward appearances. It's up to you to develop an accurate perspective. Perhaps God gave you beauty according to the world's standard. Perhaps he didn't. Whether he did or not, we must realize that we are all blessed in a variety of ways, with both human attributes and spiritual gifts. One is not better than the other; instead, it is our human perspective that has changed our perception of what has value.

Many women who are attractive by current standards confess that it's both a blessing and a curse to have physical beauty. I once overheard a senior vice president of a Fortune 500 company express his surprise at a group of attractive female marketing managers, saying, "Wow, they're pretty *and* smart . . . amazing!" It can be frustrating when doors open or close because of your looks. We must realize that this probably will never change. But it's our job to change our own thinking according to the truth.

——— *Beauty and the Bible*

There are no messages in the Bible that tell us we must look beautiful or thin to honor God. However, many references are made to our innermost being and our heart. First Peter 3:3–4 says, "Your adornment must not be merely external—braiding the hair, and wearing gold jewelry, or putting on dresses; but let it be the hidden person of the heart, with the imperishable quality of a gentle and quiet spirit, which is precious in the sight of God."

There were times when God used beauty for his own purposes. For example, Esther, who was called "beautiful of form and face," was chosen among many attractive young virgins to replace Queen Vashti. (By the way, go back and read chapter 2 in the Book of Esther and you will find one of the most extensive beauty regimes of all time. It lasted for a full year and included spices, oils, and cosmetics!) While Esther's beauty opened doors for her, it was not her greatest strength. It was her character and love for her people that is most memorable. She was willing to die for them. You may recall reading the verse in Esther 4:14 when her uncle, Mordecai, exclaims, "And who knows whether you have not attained royalty for such a time as this?" as Esther bravely goes before the king unannounced, declaring, "If I perish, I perish." Whatever the current societal view, I think the author of Proverbs 11:22 put beauty in perspective when he wrote, "As a ring of gold in a swine's snout, so is a beautiful woman who lacks discretion."

In the movie *Forest Gump*, Forest would reply to those who became aware of his limited mental capacity with the comment, "Stupid is as stupid does." His mother had taught him a healthy perspective. He had learned that while he had limitations intellectually, he could still make choices and take action based on core values.

As women living in a society that puts too much emphasis on outward beauty, we would do well to rewrite that response to: "Beauty is as beauty does." In other words, beauty is only as appealing as the underlying values and character of the person who wears the outward gift. I think that is what the writer of Proverbs 11:22 had in mind.

If we believe the lie that we are less if our beauty doesn't fall into a certain category, we doom ourselves to live a life constrained by the world's standards. Earlier, I shared my painful experience of dealing with my husband's brief infidelity. It would have been very easy to feel insecure and inadequate physically. He had been attracted to another woman. On top of that, he is seven years younger than me. And the woman he had the affair with was about ten years younger. I could have assumed that I was inferior to her because of my age. I could have assumed that she was more beautiful or appealing to him. But what good would that do me? Fortunately, my identity was secure enough to move beyond that fear. And fortunately, Lew and I were both willing to submit to God's plan for our lives and move forward.

Yet I sincerely believe I could have accepted myself and found security in Christ even if Lew had chosen to reject me and walk away. The journey would have been more difficult, the pain more intense, but truth can prevail and sustain us when we embrace it fully. Shortly after my marital challenges, God allowed me to see firsthand the incredible power that internal strength and beauty can play when we are secure in our identity despite our outward appearance.

——— *Inner Beauty*

My personal paradigm shift occurred at a speakers' conference sponsored by Florence Littauer's organization, CLASS (Christian Leaders, Authors, and Speakers Seminars). The conference's purpose was to help both seasoned and aspiring communicators fine-tune their skills. During the three days there, we were required to break into small groups and make several different presentations. As my group gathered, a woman in her thirties approached in a wheelchair. She had lost both her legs and also wore coverings on her partially amputated hands. Her face looked as if she had lost all the muscle, and her cheekbones and nose stuck out prominently from her frail skin.

My first thought was, "Oh, my, she's in our group. Is she going to be presenting?" It was not a prejudice on my part. Having been a registered nurse for years, I had seen many disturbing physical images. What surprised me was that someone in her condition would have the courage and strength of character to become a public speaker.

At first it was difficult to look at her without noticing her deformity. I was distracted by her wheelchair and the difficulty she had trying to finger through her note cards. But by the end of our three days together, I only saw one thing. I saw a beautiful and witty woman with a sparkle in her eyes and a warm and compelling message to tell. She had so much to say and so much to give that her beauty shone through.

What if I had been that woman? I wonder if I would have the strength of character and depth to rise above my physical limitations and shine through as a beautiful woman. I am sure you have met beautiful people in your life. Some are beautiful inside and out. Others are outwardly attractive, yet as you get to know them, you realize they are so self-absorbed that you no longer feel drawn to them.

Have you ever wondered how you will feel about yourself if or when your appearance meets your ideal standards? Do you think you can ever be completely satisfied? These are important questions to explore. Join me in one more imaginary experience that I believe will help you identify exactly how you feel about your body size and shape today.

— What If?

In this exercise, I would like you to imagine that a clear, odorless gas is entering the room you are in right now. It will not hurt you, but it does have one profound effect. When you breathe it, your body will be locked in at your current size and shape for the rest of your life. No matter what you do, you are stuck where you are today. How does that make you feel? Are you elated? Are you frustrated? Are you devastated? Explore for a moment how you feel and why. The answers will give you insight into how important your appearance is to you and how you view the future if you never change.

This is the most important point: Today is all you have for certain. Now is the moment you live in. Not yesterday and not tomorrow. If you feel devastated by the possibility of never changing, you will be unable to live fully in this moment. This is not to say that you should not desire improvement or make purposeful efforts to change. Rather it is to say that all future objectives must be balanced with a healthy perspective of who you are. To do otherwise minimizes your ability to celebrate and live in the moment.

I love Psalm 118:24, which says, "This is the day which the LORD has made; let us rejoice and be glad in it." In all areas of life, despite our weaknesses, we need to live in the moment, realizing that we never completely "arrive" in any area of life this side of heaven.

I challenge you to surrender your current self-image to God and ask him to help you identify the lies you believe. Then replace those lies with truths from God's Word. Imagine if you had no access to television, movies, or magazines for a full year. Instead, imagine that you were deluged with images of how God sees you. Your perspective of your own beauty would change dramatically.

So spend time each day in the arms of your heavenly Father, asking him to help you see yourself accurately. Surrender your insecurities and frustrations to him. Choose to walk in the confidence of who you are in Christ.

— 8
—— you are
— what you think

Do not be conformed to this world, but be transformed by the
renewing of your mind.

Romans 12:2

What do you say when you talk to yourself? Pay close attention.
You may just learn something very important. Have you ever
made comments like the ones below?

I'm so fat and ugly.
I know God loves me.
I just hate myself!
I've decided to change my lifestyle.
I'm out of control.
I'm in control of my choices.
I deserve this chocolate.
I think I can do it.

I'm so stressed.

Why am I so depressed?

I won't give up.

I can't do it.

I believe God will help me.

I'm such a failure.

What's wrong with me?

I understand what I'm doing wrong.

— The Soul

These statements reflect a mix of both thoughts and feelings. And that is exactly what the soul is—a blend of both mind and emotion. Our brain stores information. With our intellects we think, reason, and choose how to respond to that information. Our feelings are direct responders to our thoughts. Without thought, there would be no feeling in the emotional sense. So to change our feelings, we must change our thinking. As it says in Proverbs 23:7: "As he thinks in his mind, so is he." In essence, our most dominant thoughts "win."

Remember the character Spock on *Star Trek?* He was pure intellect without emotion. All his decisions and actions were based on logic alone. Thankfully, God has blessed us with the ability to experience the joy and excitement of life on an emotional plane. Yet every positive emotion has its negative twin. We would not be able to appreciate the height of joy without having tasted the depth of sorrow.

And so when we speak of the soul, it is both thoughts and feelings we address. Those thoughts and feelings ultimately drive us to action. The mind is the pilot of the soul. It is the control center of our entire being—our "fleshly" or temporal being, that is. And within our flesh we exercise our free will to choose our attitudes and behaviors, our beliefs and convictions. That is why it is so critical to have an identity well grounded in truth. We'll address the issue of giving up "fleshly" control and walking in the Spirit later.

— Your Mind—The Ultimate Computer

All humans are designed by their Creator to respond in specific ways, no matter what their spiritual beliefs may be. Just like the heart, liver, and kidneys are designed to perform certain vital functions, the mind also has been physiologically designed to do its job. Therefore, it is very helpful to understand how God designed this magnificent glob of gray matter and see why it does what it does! We can better appreciate the complexity of our feelings and behaviors when we understand the physiology of the human brain.

Our brain is more masterfully engineered than any man-made computer. It has been programmed to respond with consistency to an endless variety of situations. But like a computer, our brain does not place judgment on its data. True or false, it just stores it day after day, week after week, month after month, and year after year. Ultimately, we come to believe the strongest messages—those messages that have played the loudest and most frequently throughout our lives. But what if that information is wrong? Well, just imagine what would happen if someone replaced the data that is stored in the NASA computers with wrong information. The result would be disastrous. The same is true with your mind.

The Freeways of the Mind

In recent years, with the advances in medical technology, we have come to understand better how the human brain works. It seems we have an almost unlimited capacity to store information. Before birth, we begin to develop billions of neuron pathways. These are complex, microscopic circuits where all of our thoughts and experiences explode with electrical activity. And it is here where everything is stored. Some of these pathways can become physically strong and dominant because the thought or experience is frequently repeated. They become like superhighways in our mind, overriding many of the weaker pathways or less dominant thoughts.

But those neuron pathways can physically change. Old dominant pathways can shrink and become less influential when they are neglected or overridden with new messages. And smaller, weaker pathways can physically grow and become like superhighways. How? They change through repetition. I've heard it said that practice doesn't always make perfect, but it does make permanent.

From Bible scholars to the most popular modern-day motivational speakers, those who have studied human behavior know that how we think drives our choices and behavior. Though our brain functions as a storage center for information, God has also given us the ability to think, reason, and apply knowledge. He has in effect given us stewardship of our minds and, as a result, our souls. I love what Bob George says in his book *Classic Christianity:* "People are in bondage to their erroneous beliefs and it moves them into emotional and physical bondage."[1]

This is a powerful truth that can change your life for the better or for the worse. There is no permanent way to change your behavior without first changing your mind. That is why diets don't work. All the change is external. And when the diet is over, 99 percent of people revert back to old behaviors.

—— *Garbage In . . . Garbage Out! Good Stuff In . . . Good Stuff Out!*

From our simplest habits to our most destructive behaviors, our actions are a direct result of our mental programming. Both psychologists and biblical scholars agree that it is almost impossible for individuals to behave inconsistently with what they really believe about themselves. Your mind will naturally go in the direction of your most prevalent thoughts. Do you keep hitting the same lifestyle speed bumps or brick walls? Then it's time to tune in to what your thinking is doing to your life! If you don't like who you are, don't just change your behavior—change your thoughts. It may feel awkward at first, as if you're lying to yourself. But your brain doesn't know the difference. At a point, it will respond to that dominant message as if it were true.

Think of your mind as if it were a bucket filled with oil and water. Imagine that the clean, fresh water is good, positive truth and that the dirty, slimy oil floating on the top is all the negative information we receive daily from others or ourselves. Unfortunately, about 75 percent of what we receive on a daily basis is negative, and soon our minds are overflowing with oily sludge or negative thinking. But imagine if we purposely poured new, fresh truths into our minds. As the oil floats to the top of our bucket, the fresh water starts to displace it. Out spills the oil or, in this case, our old negative thoughts.

Now, of course, this is an oversimplified version of what is really happening. But I'm sure you get the picture. It's also good to remember that our minds tend to be leaky buckets. Once they are full of good information, we cannot stop infusing them with truth. They need a daily dose to counteract all the garbage coming at us!

Listen to yourself when you look in the mirror each morning. What words do you express as you resolve to lose that excess weight? How do you describe your body, your fitness, your energy, your self-control? If you keep telling yourself that you're fat and you hate exercise, you'll continue to believe it. Those beliefs will sabotage your ability to make lasting change. Like me, you've probably struggled to change old habits. You resolve to be successful this time. But how can you be successful when you've been programmed to fail? Experts agree that it takes twenty-one days even to begin breaking an old habit. It takes at least as long to form a new one. Yet on average, people can only stick to New Year's resolutions for seventeen days. No wonder they fail.

Perhaps you're trying to shed that final ten, twenty, or thirty pounds of body fat. Or maybe you've struggled for years to overcome a food addiction or an aversion to exercise. Before you have another go at it, try a more permanent approach. Try changing your mind before you change your behavior.

— Building New Pathways

Remember those neuron pathways we were just talking about? We now understand why behavioral psychologists have been saying that it takes twenty-one days to change a habit. Doctors can actually detect microscopic changes in the brain's neuron pathways after about twenty-one days of any message being repeated. The brain begins to change physiologically.

Now, don't get too excited. The change is just beginning at twenty-one days. You must maintain a consistent flow of new information for any significant changes to override old dominant thoughts and their resulting behaviors. Keep focusing on the new messages until the changes become deeply etched in your mind. It could take many months. But imagine how it will feel to move toward your goals as if you were on automatic pilot. That's exactly what dominant messages do!

——— Renew Your Mind . . . Transform Your Body

God in his perfect wisdom has provided the answers to all of life's challenges. Getting beneath the surface and discovering our true identities in Christ requires that we believe the truths from God's Word about who we are. But sometimes we know these truths intellectually and still don't believe them. It's a good thing God has the perfect solution for this problem in his Word!

112

I was so excited the first time I read Romans 12:2, which says, "Do not be conformed to this world, but be transformed by the renewing of your mind." Wow, that sounded so good! Transformed. It's a powerful word. If our minds drive all of our emotions and behaviors, this is a profound truth we must learn to act on.

It's easy to ignore the first part of that verse. We are told not to conform to this world. What does that mean? Conforming means to comply with a set of customs or standards. But as believers, we are called to be different, set apart. Our aspirations are not to be driven by worldly standards. Easy to say . . . very hard to do.

The world is bombarding us with images. You probably can recall the old cigarette commercial where an attractive young woman flaunted, "You can never be too thin or too rich." It may sound disgusting and superficial, but if we're honest, it's easy to desire both. I have learned that the way to avoid conforming and the way to be transformed are found in practicing one simple exercise: Put truth in over and over and over, until you believe it—until that neuron pathway of truth overrides all the lies.

— God's Rx for a Healthy Mind

There are many Scriptures in the Bible that address the importance of how we think. God's prescription for renewing our minds is clearly communicated in Paul's letter to the Philippians. He outlines what we must do. Here's what he wrote:

> Whatever is true, whatever is noble, whatever is right, whatever is pure, whatever is lovely, whatever is admirable—if anything is excellent or praiseworthy—think about such things. Whatever you have learned or received or heard from me or seen in me— put it into practice. And the God of peace will be with you.
>
> Philippians 4:8–9 NIV

113

——— *Pure Thinking*

As you can see by this verse, we are told to think about excellent and praiseworthy things. There are two principles at play here. First, when we consistently dwell on the right things, our neuron pathways physiologically change in a positive and spiritually purposeful way. Second, there is incredible power in God's Word. In fact, this is what the apostle Paul says about that power:

> The Word of God is living and active and sharper than any two-edged sword, and piercing as far as the division of soul and spirit, of both joints and marrow, and able to judge the thoughts and intentions of the heart.
>
> Hebrews 4:12

The Word actually divides our soul and spirit! And that sharp, two-edged sword is not some long blade used against our enemies. In this case, it is a short, surgical-type knife that we turn on ourselves. Yes, turn the truth of God's Word on yourself, and it will divide the truth from the lies. His Word will help you judge the thoughts and intentions of your heart. His Word will change your mind and ultimately change your life.

As I shared with you in chapter 3, my severe panic attacks as a young woman motivated me toward a relentless journey to find truth. During those years of internal struggle, I often doubted I would ever be free of the daily, paralyzing fear that seemed to permeate my life.

In retrospect, it is easy to understand how my fear was perpetuating more fear. I literally could bring on an attack simply by worrying about having one. It was as if someone or something was in control of my mind. And some days I was sure I was going to lose it completely.

In public, I always feared that I would make a fool of myself by becoming panicky and acting strangely. I was certain I would get in an accident while driving my car. I became overwhelmed and had to run out of crowded theaters or malls. Many days I could barely leave the house. And this fear was the catalyst that launched me on a mission to know if there was really a God and to find out if he could help me.

I had one big problem. I didn't know exactly how to "connect" with God. I was throwing up desperate pleas (better known as prayers). But how could I be sure they were even getting delivered? I thought about going to church. But how could I confirm if God knew I was there? I needed someone to help me understand how to reach out to him.

There was only one woman in my life that seemed to know God. She was one of those people who really look you in the eye and listen when you're speaking. She had what I call "smiling eyes," those premature wrinkles that come from smiling all the time. There was something special about Tonette, and it wasn't just happiness and kindness. She seemed to have something I needed much more than those things . . . peace.

I didn't want the kind of "peace" I got from taking a tranquilizer like Valium. I wanted a lasting peace that would allow me to get back to the business of living. I was seeking truth— and I found it. Tonette introduced me to my Savior, Jesus Christ.

Of course, I was hoping that he would simply heal me on the spot of all my fears and obsessions with food and my body. He didn't. He did something much more profound. He taught me how to be transformed by the renewing of my mind.

Tonette helped me dig into God's Word. And I was so hungry for answers that I could hardly set my Bible down. One day while reading, I ran across a verse that made me catch my breath. I felt as if it were written just for me. The verse is 2 Timothy 1:7, and it says: "For God has not given us a spirit of fear, but of power and of love and of a sound mind." I didn't fully comprehend at the time that Paul was giving Timothy encouragement to share the gospel boldly. Nevertheless, I believe this Scripture is applicable to us on many levels. For me, it became a lifeline of hope.

Every time I sensed a panic attack brewing, I would say the verse. I personalized it and said, "For God has not given ME a spirit of fear, but of power and of love and of a sound mind." I must have repeated those words thirty or forty times each day for the next six months. Sometimes, in times of extreme terror, I would sing them at the top of my lungs.

At the same time, I began reminding myself of other realities. Each time I felt anxious, I would tell myself that God was with me and that he had never let me die or "fall off the edge" before. And even if I did die, at least I finally knew where I was going! Over the course of the next nine months, my episodes became less intense and less frequent. At the end of one year, they occurred less than once per month and quickly subsided. Oh, the power of truth to transform us through the renewing of our minds!

—— *Positive Modeling*

Most experts agree that we learn and ultimately change in three ways: first by observation, second by imitation, and third by repetition. About 90 percent of what we do becomes reflex or habit. That's the way we are mentally programmed by God. So once we know what is true and good, it's time to find a healthy role model to follow.

You know those people who seem to be born with motivation? How do you think they got that way? Well, they probably had the incredible advantage of having excellent role models. Like with our minds, where the most dominant thought wins, the most dominant people also have a profound influence. In fact, we become like the people we spend the most time with. Of course, this truth can have both positive and negative results. You see it every day in the lives of teenagers. One day they are on track and tow-

> "If you can't be a good example, then you'll just have to serve as a horrible warning!"
>
> Catherine Aird

ing the line. The next day, they seem like strangers. What happened? Take a look at their friends and role models to get a good clue.

You may desire to have a model-like body, but have you ever really observed the lifestyle of a fashion model? The "perfect" model is airbrushed and dysfunctional. Obviously, most are not healthy examples to imitate. Design in your mind not only how you want to look and feel one year from now but also what your healthy lifestyle will be like.

Friends and coworkers with similar goals can be a great source of encouragement and support. Team up and provide some accountability to one another. Find ways to motivate your partner to hang in there. Make it a priority to take one or more of the following steps to develop powerful modeling in your life:

- Develop meaningful connections with quality people.
- Watch healthy people deal with life issues and use them as your models.
- Seek godly counsel before setting goals or taking action.
- Set boundaries with unhealthy people and limit time with them.
- Live as if you were the ultimate model for those people in your life.

No single person can ever be the perfect model for you in every area, since there is no perfect person apart from Christ. Yet Paul had enough confidence in his spiritual leadership that he could tell the Philippians to follow his lead and practice those things they had seen and heard. Find an excellent role model, mentor, or motivator and spend time with that person. If you can't identify a "live" person, go to books, videos, or other sources. It's important to choose someone who walks the talk. Make sure the lifestyle they live is healthy and practical.

—— *Practiced Obedience*

I would like to say to you, "Whatever you read, whatever I show you about living and thinking healthfully, practice these things." While I cannot, like Paul, tell my readers to follow me without restraint in every area of life, I do believe that in the lifestyle arena, I have found truth and practices that glorify God and result in healthy minds and bodies for those who choose to observe, imitate, and practice what I teach.

Observe

As you begin to work on changing your lifestyle, take time to examine the daily habits and activities of people who are healthy role models. Observe both their attitudes and behaviors concerning food, exercise, and health. You may find one person who is an excellent role model in the area of fitness, but perhaps their attitude and behaviors in the nutritional area are not worth following. Ask yourself this question: "Would I be content and honor God if I were to act like this person in this particular area?" If the answer is yes, then take the next step. Begin to imitate them.

Imitate

Paul told the Philippians to put into practice all they had received, heard, and seen from him. He also wrote in 1 Corinthians: "Be imitators of me, just as I also am of Christ" (11:1). And: "Therefore I exhort you, be imitators of me" (4:16).

Whether your role model is a real person or one you have created, begin acting like that person. Try to think, behave, eat, live, and play as he or she would. At first it may feel awkward and unnatural. Do it anyway. The first time I went snow skiing, I felt like a complete klutz skiing behind all my more experienced friends. It was a humbling experience. But after a few days, I was not only upright more often than down, I was actually having fun. Even with simple physical activities, our brain must get "synced" with our muscles in what is referred to as "muscle memory." Until those new neuron pathways are physically established, we struggle with the new movement. Neuron pathways must be developed every time we initiate new behavior. You can see this most dramatically by observing miraculous daily changes that occur in very young children. Toddlers don't give up and refuse to learn to walk because it is difficult. They just keep on trying. Soon they are running all over the house. How? They keep doing it until they get it right.

Repeat

Practice imitation repeatedly. It is at this stage that you begin to internalize the changes. The longer you practice a new behavior, the easier it becomes. Remember what I said about your neuron pathways. They don't even begin to change for about twenty-one days. Therefore, you must exercise a certain level of personal discipline before you actually sense any internal changes. Whatever you do repetitively will become locked in. Be very careful about what you think, say, or do on a regular basis.

We all demonstrate the power of repetition in the things we seem to do on "automatic pilot." Without even thinking, we revert back to what we've done most often, sometimes to our own dismay. Have you ever planned to make a quick stop on the way home from somewhere and gotten distracted? Before you know it, you're pulling into the driveway and can't even remember driving there! Without conscious and deliberate effort, our minds revert to the strongest programs. If our programs are unhealthy or ungodly, we need to change them.

Self-Talk

While gaining truth from God's Word is the most important step toward a renewed mind, we can take many practical steps to transform our thinking and ultimately change our behavior by addressing the thoughts and attitudes that are tripping us up.

Just as I used Scripture to change my thinking about my panic attacks, we can also change our thinking about anything by giving ourselves new, healthier messages.

One of the most effective ways to change your thinking is to get in tune with your "self-talk." That may sound like some kind of New Age technique for self-actualization. It's not. We all talk to ourselves. Unfortunately, most of us aren't paying attention to what we are saying in the privacy of our own minds. That's a mistake. Those silent, ongoing conversations are a huge part of our autopilot programming.

In his book *The Healing Power of the Christian Mind,* Dr. William Backus comments on the subject of self-talk.

As a clinical psychologist and pastor, I've been aware for decades how dark depressive thoughts and negative self-talk create more emotional problems than the actual events that trigger our emotions. Self-talk refers to the way we mentally process events—that is, how we interpret things that happen to us. That's why it's important to understand how our self-talk—those statements we make to ourselves—form our emotions: powerful feelings like fear, anger or worry.

Today, I am convinced that strengthening your spirit with bold, encouraging, life-giving truths that are revealed in the Bible—God's Word—will help you move toward physical wholeness and overall well-being. The Spirit communicates with your mind and your mind communicates with your body. The truth has a positive impact on our bodies when it is believed and when it is allowed to change our state of heart—that is, our moods and character.[2]

I also agree with Dr. Backus's cautions to differentiate between the miraculous hand of God and using our God-given abilities to apply deep truths to our lives in profound ways. As he puts it: "A miracle is entirely an act of God. Creating an inner climate that fosters health, on the other hand, involves our own efforts, things we can learn to do to help ourselves."[3]

Behavioral psychologist Dr. Shad Helmstetter dramatically demonstrated the principles of healthy self-talk in his own life. He had been studying the impact of how people talk to themselves in his research working with top athletes. He decided to experiment on himself and address his own challenges with losing weight.

The doctor created his own audiotape full of healthful messages about eating well and becoming more active. On the tape he told himself things such as, "I love exercise. I am in control of my eating, and I enjoy healthy foods." Each morning as he shaved at his bathroom sink, he would play his tape on a cassette player. Over the course of many months he shed fifty-eight pounds! Interestingly, his wife, who was getting ready at the other sink, also lost weight, and it wasn't even her tape! He proved for himself the truth of how the brain is designed—the most dominant thought will ultimately drive our behavior.

Positive self-talk is something you should engage in daily. Changing your mind requires a consistent supply of powerful messages. You are personally responsible to take control and ensure the regular delivery of those messages. If you don't choose to infuse transforming truths into your mind, you are surrendering control to your old lies or the negative influence of the world.

There is also a huge difference between knowing something and truly believing it. As William Backus says, "You can identify certain foods and 'believe' they exist and in fact can nourish you, but they do not until you eat them. Like real food, truthful ideas are those that feed the soul with a healthful and true picture of reality."[4]

— Setting Godly Goals

We cannot simply fix our minds on a goal and "believe to achieve." While the human capacity for change and achievement is great and few people ever maximize their potential, we still have certain inborn or circumstantial constraints. It would be absolutely ridiculous to aspire to be a professional basketball player in the NBA if you were only five foot three inches tall. The objective is to seek godly *and* realistic goals. That goes for your body as well. Pray that God will help you see your best body size and shape from his perspective. Then set your goals. In Psalm 37:4 we are told to delight in the Lord, and he will give us the desires of our heart. The point is that our desires will be his when we are delighting in him!

—— *The "One Thing"*

I believe that the most important "one thing" you can do to change any habit or behavior is to change your thinking. All the knowledge in the world is worthless if you don't believe it and apply it. But as I've already said, all your actions, habits, and behaviors are a direct result of what you truly believe. If you want to act differently, you must think differently. This one truth can transform your life in many profound ways. It's up to you.

I hope by now you are motivated to take action. Nothing will happen unless you do. Following are some specific exercises you can practice to change your self-talk. Incorporate one or more of these practices every day if you are serious about changing from the inside out. Okay, it's time to do something. It's time to take simple, daily, repetitive . . . ACTION!

—— *Identify the Lies*

Remember when you were a little kid and you'd get caught doing something wrong? Each time you were "discovered" and suffered the consequences, you became more aware of what you were doing the next time. Become aggressive at "catching yourself" in negative self-talk. Imagine clapping your hands together right in front of your nose and yelling, "Stop it!"

If you're serious about change in any area of your life, make a decision today. Identify your lies and replace them with new, healthy truths on a daily basis. Pray that God will reveal your misconceptions. Study the Word to find relevant truths that will counteract your lies, much like I did when I had my panic attacks.

Once you identify the negative "tapes" that are playing in your head, take one step farther and reverse that message. What is the positive message you choose to believe instead? Write it down and repeat it each time you catch yourself having that negative thought. Don't stop this exercise until you fully believe the new message. It may take time, but it is worth the investment because it can powerfully change your life.

—— *Change Your Lifestyle Programming*

Be honest with yourself. What's the real reason for your personal lifestyle challenges? Why do you lack motivation or commitment? What are the lies you believe? What new messages do you need to replace those lies? Take a few moments to consider and write down a response to the two statements below. Also, look at the examples that follow.

The lies I believe:
1.
2.
3.

The truths I desire to believe:
1.
2.
3.

Old negative message: I blew it again. I'll never lose weight!

123

New healthy message:	That was a great dessert. Now I can resist sweets even better. I think I'll go for a walk and burn some extra calories.
Old negative message:	I always end up quitting and never reach my goals.
New healthy message:	I'm not quitting. With God's help, I can reach my goals.
Old negative message:	I'm addicted to chocolate.
New healthy message:	I'm in control of every bite that goes into my mouth.
Old negative message:	I hate to exercise, and besides, I don't have time.
New healthy message:	I'll make time to exercise and love it!

—— Customize Your Self-Talk

Work on your new messages. Make sure you are using Scripture correctly within its appropriate context. Be sure other messages you have written are in harmony with the Word. And imagine how your life would change if you *really* believed those new truths. Do you suppose you would think and act differently if you repeated them several times a day for a full year? If the answer is yes, then do it! Read them, memorize them, repeat them until you feel as if your new, healthier lifestyle is now on automatic pilot.

Try some trigger talk. Now I'm not talking about a conversation with Roy Rogers's faithful steed or some new form of "horse whispering." Trigger talk is a useful technique that will prompt you to repeat your customized self-talk several times each day. This is how it works: Identify an activity you engage in one or more times each day, such as driving, looking at your watch, showering, or using the rest room. Use these events as "triggers" to remind you to repeat your new messages.

For example, every time you turn the key to start your car, repeat your Scripture or new statement. I call one of my most favorite triggers "potty talk." While most of us think of potty talk as a child or even an adult using bad language, I think of it as using our time in the bathroom as a trigger to change our thinking—thus, the name "potty talk." It makes sense. We all must use the bathroom several times each day. Most of us rarely are interrupted, and there's nothing else challenging our minds during this activity.

In our high-tech age, you can even use electronics to trigger you. I use my electronic day timer by scheduling it to beep at me three times a day when I want to memorize a new Scripture or get a new mental habit formed. Just imagine how your focus in life would change if three times a day you were triggered to say something like this:

"I am putting God first in my life. I am learning to love him with all my heart, soul, mind, and strength. And I am loving my family, friends, and others as myself."

Or this:

"I choose to honor God with my body. I know that his Spirit lives within me, and I am remembering to ask him for help in dealing with temptations and changing my lifestyle."

I have even created a special self-talk tape that incorporated over forty Scriptures and powerful truths to help our local clients change their unhealthy thinking patterns. It was set to music, and I recorded it in the first person, as if the individual listening were speaking directly to God. Hundreds of people have expressed that this tape was the most powerful tool in helping them transform their thinking about their appearance and habits.

— Change Is Simple, Yet Difficult

The techniques used to change your thinking are simple. Yet doing them is difficult. We are creatures of habit, and we seem to forget what we have decided to do. Find creative ways to remind yourself to use your trigger until you get into the "trigger habit." I put a Post-it note that says "Potty Talk" above the toilet paper in my bathroom. This reminds me to repeat my new messages. Or you can write your messages on the inside of your medicine cabinet, refrigerator door, or cupboard. You could put a Post-it note on your steering wheel. Do whatever it takes to remind yourself of your new activity.

Now before we go any further, grab a pen and paper and complete the following "getting started" exercise. Chances are if you save it for later, it won't happen. Set yourself apart from the crowd and ensure victory by taking some action right now!

1. Choose one or two triggers that you think will work best for you.
2. Determine what reminders you will use to trigger your triggers.
3. Write down two to four statements or Scriptures you believe will help you replace your unhealthy beliefs or thoughts.
4. Memorize them.
5. Make an effort and commitment to do this several times each day for a minimum of six months.

You will know that your trigger talk has become permanent when two things occur. First, your mind will automatically focus on that specific thought whenever you experience the trigger. Have you ever heard an old song and immediately remembered a time or place in your life? That's because the song is a powerful trigger associated with a particular time. And that's what will happen with your trigger.

126

The second thing that will validate the effectiveness of your trigger talk is that your feelings and behavior will start to change. Since your mind believes what you tell it most often, your behavior and feelings will reflect that new belief. The challenge is to practice long enough for those changes to take place.

It's up to you. In my lectures I ask people if they truly believe that giving themselves new, healthier messages can really change how they think, feel, and behave. The response is almost always a unanimous yes. Yet why is it that so few actually follow through and initiate the new behavior? I guess the simple answer is human nature. Sadly, it is easier to stay in a comfort zone of unhealthy thinking and living than to take simple steps toward a victorious life.

What will ensure that you are successful at changing your old thinking? You will. The bottom line is this: You must choose to change your old thinking patterns and subsequently your old habits. You must want the benefit these changes will bring (like an energetic, lean body).

Never forget the power of your thoughts. There's a quote I've heard and shared through the years that I believe sums up the power of our mind.

Watch your thoughts; they become your words.
Watch your words; they become your actions.
Watch your actions; they become your habits.
Watch your habits; they become your character.
Watch your character; it becomes your destiny.

While our ultimate destinies as believers are secured in heaven, our earthly destinies will depend on what dominates our minds. When we fill our minds with God's truth and then seek to do the right things for the right reasons, we will achieve more than renewed minds and transformed bodies. We will experience what Paul promises at the end of Philippians 4:9—that the God of peace will be with us.

127

— A Personal Lifestyle Evaluation

Hopefully you took the initial evaluations in chapter 2. Now, after reading this chapter, you may see these same questions with a little more insight. Your answers will most likely be the same for now. Change will occur as you apply these principles. Take this evaluation again and every couple months to gauge your journey toward victory! Base your answers on your most consistent behavior or attitudes in the past three months. It should take you about four to five minutes.

- **Don't** rate yourself based on any changes you've made in the last four to six weeks.
- **Do** rate yourself based on your first impression and move on.
- **Don't** go back and readjust your answers if you don't like the score.
- **Do** remember . . . this is a reality check. Just face the truth and move on.

Are you ready? Grab a pencil and be completely honest. No one has to see the results but you!

—— *Lifestyle Evaluation—Perspective/Motivation*

Based on the last three months, please rate yourself (0–Almost never; 1–Sometimes; 2–Often; 3–Always).

_____ I see myself as a fully accepted and loved child of God.

_____ My choices and actions are made based on my relationship to Christ.

_____ I am thankful for the body God has given me.

_____ I honor God with my lifestyle habits.

_____ I take responsibility for my body's size, shape, and health.

_____ My attitude is this: I am not my behavior. I am complete in Christ.

_____ I surrender my weaknesses to God and rely on his strength for the moment.

_____ My personal goals are realistic and honor God.

_____ I take realistic steps toward my goals each day.

_____ I know that with God's help, I can have a lean, healthy body.

_____ I am aware of the lies I believe about my body, looks, and health.

_____ I recognize and choose not to accept this negative thinking.

_____ I renew my mind with God's truth each day.

_____ I am a work in progress, and God delights in each good step I take.

_____ Each day, I choose to submit my body, mind, and spirit to God.

_____ I pray daily for God's strength and power to walk in the Spirit and not fulfill the desires of my flesh.

_____ Add the total of all scores.

Scoring

40–48 Excellent! You have a godly perspective.

31–39 Good. Your perspective usually is working for you.

22–30 Fair. It's time to get a new focus . . . the truth!

< 21 Alert! Alert! Change your perspective now!

— Perspective/Healthy Thinking Menu

—— *The "One Thing"*

Do you think and live as if your relationship with God is your highest priority?

How can you make intimacy with the Lord your greatest desire?

What do you need to do to make this a reality?

Do you need more time . . .

In the Word? In prayer? In meditation? In worship?

Write it down!

—— *Attitudes*

Do you have any unhealthy attitudes?

What new attitude will you focus on instead?

Know your identity in Christ.

Develop a body image in sync with God's perspective of you.

Develop a "small steps" perspective . . . small stuff counts and adds up!

—— *Self-Talk*

Identify your negative messages.

Replace them with truth, using: ☐ Index cards ☐ Tapes ☐ Trigger talk

—— *People Power*

Role models: Who are you modeling your lifestyle after?

Spiritual mentors: Who are you modeling your spiritual walk after?

Positive motivators: Who can help you along the way?

Do you need a personal coach or an exercise or accountability partner?

—— *Goals*

What are your goals?
Do they honor God?
Do you have realistic expectations?
Are you submitting and surrendering them to God?
Now . . . write them down!

> Do not be conformed to this world, but be transformed by the renewing of your mind.
>
> Romans 12:2

—— *Using Other Resources*

Journal for deeper insights.

— Design Your Lifestyle

My Perspective/Healthy Thinking Recipe

Priority	Action
#1 _____	_____
	_____
	_____
#2 _____	_____
	_____
	_____
#3 _____	_____
	_____
	_____
#4 _____	_____
	_____
	_____

— 9

—— the battle
— of the flesh

Jenny remembered how great it felt to slip into her smallest jeans. She loved how she looked with her shirt tucked in. Her stomach was flat. Her waist was small. What a rush to see the reflection in the three-way mirror and realize it was really her! She loved that old phrase she had learned at a weight-management meeting: "Thin feels better than this food tastes." Jenny was absolutely convinced that she would never give in to her old bad habits. It just felt too good to be thin.

That was two years ago. Jenny enjoyed the marvelous feeling for a fleeting ten months. Then over the next fourteen months, she returned one size at a time back to the "original" Jenny. What happened? Why was it so hard to keep the weight off? It was almost more defeating to have lost and gained the weight back than never to have lost it at all. She felt like a complete failure.

Have you ever wondered why you do the things you do? Does it sometimes seem like you have no control over your emotions or behavior? Do you ever feel like you are waging a war?

We *are* in a battle—with ourselves. We are often our most formidable enemy. But where will we find victory? Most of us have tried the route of self-discipline and commitment over and over. And we have failed—over and over.

Our minds control our souls. And as we learned earlier, we can change our minds and ultimately our behavior. But if we do that using our own human strength, we are missing an essential element of the Christian walk. As believers, we have God as our ultimate power source for living in true victory. Yet despite the fact that we have access to that power, we often choose to live our lives "unplugged."

You probably own a power vacuum. Ever tried to vacuum your rug without plugging the appliance in or turning it on? Nothing happens. You can push it around with a fair amount of effort, but the carpet remains the same. You may as well just get out a broom, which will produce minimal results.

That's how our lives are when we operate on our own power. I should know. For many years I lived what I would describe as being "saved without victory." I knew that Christ had paid the price for my sin and had secured my eternity in heaven, but in my daily life, there was very little victory. Like Jenny, I sometimes wondered why I was living in such utter defeat.

— The Battle Rages On

From dawn till dusk I battled my secret demon—food. And each hour, I struggled with conflicting desires. I wanted to be lean, healthy, and in control of my appetite. I also wanted to eat everything in sight. Every day I made a firm resolve to control my outrageous behavior. I planned each meal and thought of strategies to avoid my eating triggers, but I rarely succeeded in making it through one day without a binge. I constantly asked myself, "What is wrong with me? Why am I so weak?" One night, I woke myself up talking in my sleep. I was sobbing and saying over and over, "You . . . just . . . eat when you're hungry! Eat when you're hungry!" Year after year I struggled. Year after year I lost the battle. In my second year of college, I would often binge and purge up to five times a day. It seemed as if my entire life was spinning out of control. Over time, I began to doubt if there was any hope for me.

What is it that drives us to do that which we don't really want to do? How is it we give in again and again to temptations that seem out of our control? Everyone battles at some point with a particular area of temptation or sin. I think Paul describes this constant war of the flesh perfectly in Romans 7:15: "For what I am doing, I do not understand; for I am not practicing what I would like to do, but I am doing the very thing I hate."

If the great apostle Paul struggled, what makes us think we are any different? But should this fact make us throw in the towel? Absolutely not! I think this Scripture helps us understand an important reality—all believers struggle with a battle of the flesh. Paul continues in verses 18–20:

> For I know that nothing good dwells in me, that is, in my flesh; for the willing is present in me, but the doing of the good is not. For the good that I want, I do not do, but I practice the very evil that I do not want. But if I am doing the very thing I do not want, I am no longer the one doing it, but sin which dwells in me.

Does that sound like Paul is making excuses for his behavior? He isn't. He's stating a fact. Sin continued to be a challenge for him, and it continues to be a challenge for us. But the difference between a saint and a sinner is that the saint (those who believe their salvation is found only through Christ's death, burial, and resurrection) has the option to walk in the Spirit. Until we are in Christ, our spirits are dead, and we have only one option—to walk in the flesh.

This is not to say that all who walk in the flesh are sinning. They are simply living under their own personal power. There are many "good" people in the world who are not believers. They volunteer their time and monies to worthwhile charities. They invest quality moments with their children. They lead exemplary lives—all on their own steam. They may make good and moral choices or poor and immoral choices. Either way, it is simply a human choice. But as children of God, we have the Spirit of God living within us. Not only are we forgiven and justified through the blood of Christ, we are also indwelt with the Holy Spirit. We now have supernatural power over our propensity to sin. Nevertheless, on a moment-to-moment basis, the saint is still capable of giving in to the flesh and sometimes giving in to sin. Paul clarifies more in verses 21–24:

> I find then the principle that evil is present in me, the one who wants to do good. For I joyfully concur with the law of God in the inner man, but I see a different law in the members of my body, waging war against the law of my mind and making me a prisoner of the law of sin which is in my members. Wretched man that I am! Who will set me free from the body of this death?

Is Paul's continued sin putting his salvation at risk? No! The death he speaks of is a deadening of his soul and a diminished fellowship with the Lord. So Paul looks to the only source of strength, power, and forgiveness—our Lord and Savior Jesus Christ—and exclaims:

> Thanks be to God through Jesus Christ our Lord! So then, on the one hand I myself with my mind am serving the law of God, but on the other, with my flesh the law of sin. Therefore, there is now no condemnation for those who are in Christ Jesus. For the law of the Spirit of life in Christ Jesus has set you free from the law of sin and of death.
>
> Romans 7:25; 8:1–2

In other words, our sins no longer judicially condemn us. As believers, we are free from eternal condemnation—our eternity is secure in heaven. And in this temporal life, we are free to choose which path we will walk each moment of each day . . . the path of the flesh or the path of the Spirit. The question is: How do we stay on the path of the Spirit and realize absolute power and victory right now?

— Choosing Your Path

Imagine for a moment opening up your door tomorrow morning and discovering two distinctly paved and landscaped paths extending from your front porch. One is beautiful and enticing. Its smooth stones and breathtaking landscaping draw you in. You are certain it will bring you immediate pleasure and reward. The other is a much narrower path, and you cannot see beyond more than a few steps. It seems less attractive and compelling. It requires that you trust the one who has prepared the way for you. Which will you choose?

—— *The Path of Least Resistance*

The first is the path of the world, the one that draws your flesh by promising to meet your immediate needs. It seems like the right choice. It "feels" right. Sometimes, the path of the world is simply the road you travel on your own steam. It doesn't mean that everything you do in the flesh is bad or immoral. It is simply done under your own power.

Even works of ministry can be done "in the flesh." Explore your motives. Are you doing acts of service for the glory of God or for your own gratification? Do you say yes to volunteer work because you know it makes you look good? Do you get involved in some ministries because you think it will earn you points with God? God isn't impressed. I believe he involves us in the work of ministry to bless us. He could do it all without us but chooses not to.

The Path of Self-Discipline

We can produce good things in the flesh; we can use our own self-discipline and personal motivations to accomplish our personal goals. There is a small population of people who actually lose weight and keep it off without any help from God. How? By using their own strength. In fact, part of your journey with me toward a healthier lifestyle will actually be taken under your own human power. There is nothing wrong with developing some new habits and behaviors using your own gumption. Yet why should we take an incomplete and self-powered route when we have something so much better available?

The Path with Real Power

When we live and act out of love for God without a thought for ourselves, this is the path of the Spirit, a path where both our motives and actions are pure. But it's tough to stay on that selfless path. That's because we can't travel it under our own power. Some would have you believe that Christians can stay on the narrow path as long as they are disciplined and committed to God. This simply is not true. The "disciplined" walk is simply a "flesh walk" that looks spiritual.

Walking with God is not a matter of discipline and commitment; it is a matter of surrender. We'll discuss how to surrender and live under the power of the Spirit a little later. But first, let's dig a little deeper into God's Word and see what more it has to say about the battle that is raging—the battle we so desperately desire to win.

We receive more teaching about this subject in Galatians 5:16, where Paul writes: "But I say, walk by the Spirit, and you will not carry out the desire of the flesh." Now if walking by the Spirit were an automatic response to being born again, Paul wouldn't have to tell us to do it! And if it were impossible to do, he wouldn't even exhort us to try. Yet he reminds us of the intensity of the struggle as he continues in verse 17: "For the flesh sets its desire against the Spirit, and the Spirit against the flesh; for these are in opposition to one another, so that you may not do the things that you please." It is obvious that we are in the same battle Paul had in Romans 7. All believers will battle. If they say they don't, they are lying.

— Saved and Sinning?

This is one of the most challenging paradoxes of the Christian walk—believers can sin and still be saved. But I've learned a profound truth found in Scripture that has helped me in understanding the dynamics of sin and repentance. Repentance means to change your mind or to reverse direction. However, there are two distinct types of repentance.

The first occurs when we, as nonbelievers, recognize and repent of three things. First, we repent of our condition as sinners, because we finally understand that no matter how "good" we are, we are not good enough. In fact, we are contaminated from birth. Second, we repent of our false view of Christ, that we did not believe he is God incarnate. And last, we repent of our false view of salvation, our belief that we could save ourselves by being good people. In Romans 3:23 Paul writes, "For all have sinned and fall short of the glory of God." This is the repentance that Jesus spoke of in Mark 1:14–15: "Jesus came into Galilee, preaching the gospel of God, and saying, 'The time is fulfilled, and the kingdom of God is at hand; repent and believe in the gospel.'"

The second form of repentance is one that we as believers will experience many times in this journey of life as we struggle and give in to the temptations of the flesh. God in his awesome grace has saved us from our sins. By faith in Christ, we are set free from condemnation and are eternally justified and secured as children of God. Yet even though we are saints, we often allow the flesh to win out. In order to restore full intimacy with the Lord, we must repent of specific sins. We must acknowledge our transgressions and turn and walk the other way.

In his book *Classic Christianity*, Bob George uses a most powerful analogy to illustrate our ability to choose between our fleshly (often sinful) desires and the great riches we receive when we walk in the Spirit. He shares a story of a restaurant owner who finds a starving, homeless beggar digging through the dumpster behind his restaurant, looking for scraps of food. The man invites the beggar in and tells him that he can eat there every day and choose anything he wants. The beggar can scarcely believe his eyes as he looks at all the incredibly delicious food. He asks, "I can have anything?" The restaurant owner nods his head. "Yes, absolutely anything," he replies. Slowly, with a gleam in his eye, the beggar asks, "Can I eat some garbage?"[1]

As Bob George concludes, that is exactly what we choose to do when we choose sin. God has given us the liberty of choice—his riches or the world's pleasures. Why is it we so often choose the garbage?

Before you get frustrated and give up, Paul delivers some encouraging news in Galatians: "But the fruit of the Spirit is love, joy, peace, patience, kindness, goodness, faithfulness, gentleness, self-control; against such things there is no law" (Gal. 5:22–23).

Perspectives on Bearing Fruit

Wow. Wouldn't you love to have a spiritual fruit basket overflowing with all those wonderful attributes, all the time? Is that even possible? It must be, because Paul continues in verse 24: "Now those who belong to Christ Jesus have crucified the flesh with its passions and desires."

He says that we have crucified our flesh with its passions and desires. At first glance, it may seem as if this verse tells us that the battle is already won. But we know from his previous comments (and the evidence in our own lives) that this simply is not true. I think what he means is that our faith in Christ gives us the power to subjugate our self-centered worldview to a Christ-centered perspective that puts the things of God above our own fleshly desires. Notice how he continues in verse 25: "If we live by the Spirit, let us also walk by the Spirit."

When Paul speaks of living by the Spirit, he means that we have eternal life by the Spirit. Knowing this, he encourages us to be dependent upon the Spirit for living victoriously "in time" (that is now) as well. That is what he means by the term "walking by the Spirit." We have all of the Holy Spirit we will ever get when we receive Christ as our Savior. He is resident in our lives. Yet despite this truth, we often spend much of our time walking in the futility of the flesh.

——— *The Holy Spirit and Chocolate Milk*

I once had a Bible teacher describe the power of the Holy Spirit in our lives using the analogy of chocolate milk. She said to imagine squirting thick chocolate syrup into a tall glass of milk. The syrup immediately sinks to the bottom of the glass. Is the chocolate in the milk? Sure. Has it permeated the entire glass? No. It lays on the bottom, available but not activated. Grab a spoon and stir it up, and the whole glass of milk becomes chocolate.

This simple example illustrates how we can live with the Spirit of God *in* us without allowing him power *over* us. God could choose to override our wills at any time. He rarely does. He allows our frustration and sense of futility with our own efforts to bring us back to him eventually. Then we are forced to realize our own inadequacy, and we get on our knees and ask, "How do I 'stir up' your Spirit in my life and live in your power alone, Lord?"

141

God's Part

If you are a Christian, God has already given you all spiritual blessings. You have reconciliation and intimacy with him for eternity through the blood of Christ. You have the Holy Spirit and his power available to you. You have the future hope of complete sanctification and a glorified body when Christ returns. You have the truth from his Word to guide and empower your life. He's done his part. Now it's time for you to do yours.

Your Part

As I mentioned earlier, most Christians believe that leading a holy life is all about personal discipline and commitment. But we've discovered that all our human effort is still walking in the flesh, no matter how good or outwardly spiritual we are. Remember the Pharisees? They didn't impress Christ. And our human efforts don't impress him either. They are like "wood, hay and straw" to God (1 Cor. 3:12).

So what must we do to "stir up" the Spirit and walk consistently on the path God has set before us? How do we produce the fruit of the Spirit Paul spoke about in Galatians? Consistent with Paul's teaching, John gives us a clearer picture when he shares what Jesus told his disciples in the parable of the vine. Jesus says:

> "Abide in Me, and I in you. As the branch cannot bear fruit of itself unless it abides in the vine, so neither can you unless you abide in Me. I am the vine, you are the branches; he who abides in Me and I in him, he bears much fruit, for apart from Me you can do nothing."
>
> John 15:4–5

"Abide" means to stay in a given place, state, relation, or expectancy. It means to dwell, endure, remain, or stand. We all know what happens if we pull a branch off of a tree. It dies. It has no life to produce fruit. In this parable, Jesus is speaking of specific spiritual fruit—all those wonderful manifestations of walking in the Spirit Paul spoke of in Galatians. (You know, the list that ends with *self-control*.) In fact, it would appear that abiding and walking in the Spirit is the same thing. Jesus continues in John 15:7–8:

> "If you abide in Me, and My words abide in you, ask whatever you wish, and it will be done for you. My Father is glorified by this, that you bear much fruit, and so prove to be My disciples."

In the Greek, the word *abide* means to settle down and be at home. It is when we stay close to our Lord and depend on him for all our nourishment and existence. He says that when his words abide in us, we may ask whatever we wish and it will be done. So often, we focus on the "ask whatever we wish" part of that verse and neglect the most important caveat. He said *when* his Word abides in us, *then* we can ask. His words cannot abide in us unless we know what they are.

— Stay Close . . . Abide

If you are a parent or have ever cared for children, you know that they will often ask for something that is not good for them. I remember when my oldest daughter got her first two-wheel bike for Christmas. She was so excited that she could barely contain herself. She wanted to jump on it immediately and ride it down the street. The problem was that she didn't know how. She didn't understand why her father thought she would fall over and get hurt. She'd seen all the other kids riding, and it looked so easy. She soon discovered after a badly scraped knee that it was a good idea to wait for Dad. As he gently held on and walked beside her, she began to get her balance. She wanted him to stay very near, and she paid close attention to his words of instruction on how to maneuver her new bike.

That is how it is with us every day of our lives. We need to stay very close to our heavenly Father. We need to understand his words and let them give us nourishment and life. He wants us to glorify him by bearing spiritual fruit; but there are no shortcuts. There are no blessings that come ahead of abiding. If they did, then we wouldn't abide.

So if abiding in Christ means staying close to God, how do we accomplish that daily intimacy? In James 4:8 it says, "Draw near to God and He will draw near to you." Draw near to God. Submit. Abide. Stay close . . . very, very close. Hang on for dear life.

Yet even when we desire to abide in Christ, our flesh is still looking for a shortcut. We want a simple formula to follow. There are books that tell you to pray a certain prayer for thirty days and see what happens. There are services to deliver you from your strongholds, and spiritual programs that teach you how to change your circumstances.

Just like dieting, we make it all so complicated. I have found that God has made things profoundly simple. There are no new breakthroughs or spiritual secrets to uncover. He has spelled out the simplicity of abiding and living a fruitful life clearly in his Word. The key to deep spiritual victory in any dimension of our lives requires fulfilling the greatest of all commandments, which Christ told us was "Love the Lord your God with all your heart, and with all your soul, and with all your mind" (Matt. 22:37).

This commandment raises a question: How do I love God with all my being? Well, we come to love him when we learn to abide in him. When we abide in him, we naturally walk in the Spirit. I know it sounds like a never-ending circle. It is. As I've already said, the answer is simple, yet difficult.

—— *The Key: God-Obsession*

We come to know him by spending time in prayer, worship, and meditation on his Word. These are intensely personal times when we surrender our wills and spirits to him and allow his Spirit to work in our minds and hearts.

144

What do you think of when you hear the word *godliness*? I have been taught that it is equivalent to being "God-obsessed." I've been obsessed with food, with exercise, sometimes even with accomplishing good things *for* God. But wouldn't it be great to be totally obsessed *with* God every moment of every day? This is the one obsession that would be healthy and life changing. And that is our ultimate goal. To be so transformed by the truth of God's complete and powerful presence in our lives that everything else is secondary.

— The Enemy: Satan or Me?

Sometimes we get confused about whom we are battling with. Is it our own fleshly desires or is it the enemy trying to trip us up? I used to struggle with that concern. If I knew the difference, I would know how to respond, right? Then I discovered a liberating truth. It doesn't matter as much as you think. Satan's greatest tool is deception. Once we are deceived, we do the rest very well on our own.

So whether it is the enemy, our own fleshly desires, or a combination of both, the key is to prepare for battle and stand ready. Imagine if we sent our troops into the Middle East to fight terrorism without preparing them for the fight. If we waited until they got there to brief them on the enemy's tactics or to show them how to use their weapons and armor, they'd be in deep trouble. A wise soldier puts on his armor before he goes into battle. A wise Christian does so as well. Unfortunately, our battle is continuous. I would encourage you to read the sixth chapter of Ephesians, where Paul details how to "take up the full armor of God, so that you will be able to resist in the evil day, and having done everything, to stand firm" (6:13).

Without getting into another extensive study, I want to point out a couple of key truths on this subject. First, you can put on the armor of God and have great benefit even if you are only battling your own flesh. Second, Paul is reviewing key spiritual principles related to the power of truth, our security in Christ, the significance of faith, and the necessity for us to do our part—to stand firm and pray.

There are two significant things I think we need to spend more energy on as victorious believers: (1) Turning the sword of the Spirit (the Word of God) on *ourselves* so that we can be transformed by the renewing of our minds; and (2) praying at all times with great fervency and perseverance.

In the next chapter, I will address the battle of the flesh most people are way too familiar with: emotional eating. I hope you will consider the truths from this chapter as you explore practical and sometimes "fleshly" ways to address your emotional eating issues.

As I close, I'd like to pass on some "fruit" one of my clients grew as a result of going on this lifestyle journey. When I am teaching, God sometimes delivers a gift to me—allowing me to see the transformation in the hearts and minds of my lifestyle students. One day as I was gathering up my teaching materials at the end of class, I noticed a nicely formatted and printed page sitting on one of the tables. Kathy, a woman who had been battling with her weight for many years, expressed the concept of walking in the Spirit in terms of her lifestyle with these words:

Love. Love yourself enough to take care of the body God has given you. Love God enough to treat it properly.

Joy. Have joy for today because of exactly who you are right NOW. Have joy for whose you are.

Peace. Embrace the peace only God provides by fully trusting in him and his plans for you . . . peace that tells you that you will have victory.

Patience. Have patience for that victory. Remember God's perfect timing in the past and cling to that evidence for your future.

146

Kindness. Show kindness to yourself. Say positive things about yourself and don't criticize yourself when you are not eating "perfectly."

Goodness. Dwell on the goodness of the Lord and focus on the good changes you are making in your lifestyle.

Faithfulness. God is faithful, and he will give you faithfulness in your decision to make these new and healthier lifestyle changes.

Gentleness. Pamper yourself . . . no, not with tons of "comfort food" but with the gentleness and comfort that only comes from abiding in Christ.

Self-Control. Yes, you can have self-control! Call upon the powers and grace of God Almighty. He is waiting to give you strength.

If we focus on walking in the Spirit, these fruits will abound . . . and don't they sound just luscious? Besides, our body needs a good supply of "fruit" each and every day!

Part 2

The Journey
of Transformation

— 10
—— overcoming
— emotional eating

Whether, then, you eat or drink or whatever you do, do all to the glory of God.

1 Corinthians 10:31

"I bought a carrot cake last week, and most of it is still in my refrigerator!" Sharon was so excited she could hardly contain herself. "You've got to know, this is the first time this has ever happened! I've been telling myself there are no forbidden foods, that I can eat what I want, when I want to, so why eat it all now? And I'm really starting to believe it! I don't feel guilty. I feel like I'm finally in control after all these years!"

Statements like this bring tears to my eyes. After years of struggling with my own emotional eating issues, I fully under-stand the incredible sense of victory and release that comes with triumphing over an unhealthy relationship with food.

We all have different issues that drive our relationships with food. This chapter is designed to help you go beneath the surface to determine your emotional eating triggers and to develop healthy eating attitudes and skills.

Before we dig into some practical ways of dealing with the day-to-day temptation with food, let me remind you of what we've already discussed. That is, no amount of self-control or eating strategies will ever take the place of the self-control that comes from walking in the Spirit. So don't let these fleshly strategies distract you from the "one thing." Your time alone with God will always be the most important strategy for victorious living. While it's not an instant cure for the munchies, it is the ultimate cure for desiring God's glorification over your immediate gratification.

— Do You Live to Eat?

Emotional eating is just one battle of the flesh in the lifestyle arena. It requires its own chapter, because it is my observation that the large majority of women who have weight problems are also emotional eaters. Do you ever feel like you live to eat more than you eat to live? Is food a driving force in your day? Do you wish you could simply put it out of your mind and desire it only when you are physiologically hungry? So did I.

But I have great news. You *can* get there—maybe not every single hour of every single day, but more often than not. And sometimes you'll actually forget to eat. What a concept!

—— *Food on the Mind*

Think of the times when food wasn't on your mind. In times of great pain—like when you're in labor! Or times of great fear—when someone almost runs you off the road. Or times of great anxiety—when you have to give a speech in front of two hundred of your peers. Bet you weren't thinking about food during those times, eh? And of course there are times when you experience something so special that food is absolutely the last thing on your mind—like when you are walking down the aisle with your new husband.

If you think you are a miserable wretch because food seems to have so much importance in your life, don't feel too badly. You're not alone. Humans have been battling with idols of the flesh since the Garden. And just because your battle shows in extra storage tanks of unburned fuel (fat cells), don't think those who don't battle with food are exempt from their own struggles. Whether food, alcohol, materialism, pride, or some other form of lust, we all have a "pet" idol to contend with.

We can learn a lot about human nature by studying the Israelites and their appetites. Most of us have viewed Hollywood's adaptation of the great exodus from Egypt with Moses leading the way. Can you imagine the impact of seeing firsthand the kind of miracles the Israelites had experienced? First, the Spirit of the Lord passed over all the homes that had the blood of a lamb over the doorpost and spared the firstborn children. Then the Israelites saw the sea miraculously part, allowing them to escape their captors. Then the Lord went before them as a pillar of cloud by day and a pillar of fire by night to lead them toward the Promised Land. And he provided fresh water to drink and sent food from heaven called manna. Miracle after miracle, God clearly demonstrated his presence and provision. You would think the Israelites would be in awe. You would think they would be satisfied and grateful. You would think.

Yet they lost sight of their deliverance and focused on their appetites, saying:

> "Who will give us meat to eat? We remember the fish which we used to eat free in Egypt, the cucumbers and the melons and the leeks and the onions and the garlic, but now our appetite is gone. There is nothing at all to look at except this manna."
>
> Numbers 11:4–6

153

Well, at least they desired healthy food! But God was giving them all the nutrition they needed in the manna, and they were ungrateful. It didn't satisfy their appetites. They preferred being slaves in Egypt so they could gratify their palates. What they didn't realize is that they were still slaves . . . slaves to their flesh. Of course, Moses was beside himself. He hadn't asked for this. Nothing like a bunch of complainers in the wilderness to put a damper on your freedom celebration! So he called out to the Lord, asking him to provide meat or otherwise just kill him and put him out of his misery right then and there. And the Lord replied:

"Say to the people, 'Consecrate yourselves for tomorrow, and you shall eat meat; for you have wept in the ears of the LORD, saying "Oh that someone would give us meat to eat! For we were well-off in Egypt." Therefore the LORD will give you meat and you shall eat. You shall eat, not one day, nor two days, nor five days, nor ten days, nor twenty days, but a whole month, until it comes out of your nostrils and becomes loathsome to you; because you have rejected the LORD, who is among you and have wept before Him saying, "Why did we ever leave Egypt?"'"

Numbers 11:18–20

You can't miss the sarcasm in the words of the Lord. He gave them what they needed, and they rejected it. Now, he gave them what they wanted, and they would come to regret it. This is what happened:

While the meat was still between their teeth, before it was chewed, the anger of the LORD was kindled against the people, and the LORD struck the people with a very severe plague. So the name of that place was called Kibroth-hattaavah, because there they buried the people who had been greedy.

Numbers 11:33–34

Wow. I'm thankful God doesn't deal with us as harshly today. Living under grace is an incredible blessing. Yet we still pay the price for the idolatry of our fleshly desires. Paul used this example in his teaching to the Corinthians, who were struggling with all sorts of fleshly desires.

> Now these things happened as examples for us, so that we would not crave evil things as they also craved. Do not be idolaters, as some of them were; as it is written, "THE PEOPLE SAT DOWN TO EAT AND DRINK, AND STOOD UP TO PLAY."
>
> 1 Corinthians 10:6–7

What Paul is saying is that we are not to put anything above God. In the same chapter of 1 Corinthians, he continues to teach on the subject of temptation, which he ultimately relates to idolatry. He says:

> No temptation has overtaken you but such as is common to man; and God is faithful, who will not allow you to be tempted beyond what you are able, but with the temptation will provide the way of escape also, so that you will be able to endure it. Therefore, my beloved, flee from idolatry.
>
> 1 Corinthians 10:13–14

I have noticed that many Christians seem to expect that God will provide some kind of miraculous deliverance from every temptation. They expect the phone to ring and call them away from the cookie jar. I don't think so. Who exactly is forcing the cookie down their throats? I'm sorry to be so blunt, but in all my years of compulsive bingeing, not one cookie jumped into my mouth without my help! I believe the most practical way of escape is found at the end of that verse—*flee.*

Additionally, I believe that preparing for the battle before you are in the heat of it is essential. I hope you will find the following insights and exercises helpful in addressing your emotional eating issues. These are not magical cures, however. They simply are strategies for waging war until the ultimate battle of your mind is complete. That is, until you are transformed by truth, surrendered to God's power, and walking in the Spirit in this area of your life.

—— *HALT!*

Noteworthy preacher and teacher Charles Stanley did a wonderful job preaching about the battle of the flesh.[1] He warns that we need to get in tune with those things or events that play into our particular areas of weakness. He says there are four critical times when we tend to "give in" more readily to the flesh. You can remember them by the acronym and appropriate word of warning: HALT. He says those common triggers occur whenever we are:

Hungry
Angry
Lonely
Tired

I agree with Dr. Stanley. We need to be tuned into the things that take us to the edge. It is much easier to prepare for the challenge before we get there than when we are hanging on by our fingernails. Just as we discussed in the previous chapter, we need to prepare for our battles in practical ways, both spiritual and in the flesh.

—— *The Event/Food Connection*

Do you ever feel like food has the upper hand in your life? Does chocolate call your name from the dessert bar or does popcorn jump right into your arms at the movies? Food is an important part of our lives and has been since day one. Our first cries frequently were cries of hunger. Food became comfort and security for most of us in many situations throughout our lives.

At birthdays and weddings, we celebrate with special cakes and treats. Holidays have foods and traditions tied to them. Every event, like ball games, the theater, or visits to the zoo, elicits a craving for the food we associate with that particular experience. Add to that television, magazines, and all of our friends and acquaintances bombarding us with different food sensations, and we have a never-ending temptation to gorge ourselves with one treat after another. Couple this with the simple fact that food tastes great, and we have a disaster just waiting to happen. Perhaps it already has—in the form of overexpanded fat cells and clothes that just don't fit like they used to.

However, all forms of overeating do not indicate you have a dangerous relationship with food. Sometimes, we simply choose to indulge more than usual. Emotional eating is only a problem when it leads to daily habits you feel you cannot control.

— Healthy Eating

Ultimately, what we want and should have is a healthy relationship with food, where we believe the truth that we *are* in control of our choices. When life is crazy or when you're a little stressed or bored, you sometimes choose to eat for the pure pleasure of it. Whether you struggle daily or just occasionally with emotional eating issues, this chapter will help you develop a healthier relationship with food for the rest of your life.

What is a healthy relationship with food?

- Understanding that all days are not exactly the same.
- Being able to eat when you are hungry and continue until you feel comfortably satisfied. But occasionally, it is also letting yourself eat a little more than you should, just because you want to.
- Choosing to refrain from some foods because you want to improve your health or feel better.

- Knowing you can have anything you want, any time you want it, so you don't have to have it all right now.
- Enjoying and finding pleasure in food. This also means that there are times when other things distract you, and you couldn't care less.
- Knowing when enough is enough and finding other coping mechanisms in life besides food to help you through tough times.
- Being in control of your food choices, because you know you really are.

— Three Key Areas of Emotional Eating

In order to get a handle on your emotional eating, it is helpful to explore three key areas.

—— #1—Legalizing Food

Let's start with the concept of legalizing food. Most of us have been on more than a few diets in our lives, and most diets deal with restraint and an external control on food. Dieters often believe that certain foods are okay and others are forbidden. This belief creates a struggle and a conflict—a mental tug-of-war. As long as there is a struggle, there is potential for bingeing and actually eating more than normal. This all-or-nothing attitude is very self-destructive. The minute we tell ourselves we can't have something, guess what we want more than ever? (Remember the "air diet"?)

I think that as Christians we often take a legalistic stand on foods. They are either "good" or "bad." All foods have caloric value. In other words, they provide energy to the body. If all we eat are empty calories, our bodies are fueled without complete nourishment. Yet in balance we can enjoy an occasional dessert or snack just for the pleasure of it.

In the Bible we read of times of both fasting and feasting. I'm sure you've read about the fattened calves being slaughtered for a celebration, or the Promised Land being described as a land "flowing with milk and honey." God gave us many things both to sustain us and bless us. And he gave us our five senses for both protection and pleasure. It is how we use them that determines whether they become a blessing or a curse.

As believers in Christ, we are no longer under the law. Even Paul had to address believers' concerns about eating meat that previously had been sacrificed to idols. The problem was not the meat but the believers' attitudes toward the meat. Paul writes:

> All things are lawful for me, but not all things are profitable. All things are lawful for me, but I will not be mastered by anything. Food is for the stomach and the stomach is for food, but God will do away with both of them.
>
> 1 Corinthians 6:12–13

If God is going to do away with food in eternity, we'd better find much more fulfilling ways to satisfy our souls! Once again, I must remind you—this will take time. But with a surrendered heart and a focus on finding your greatest satisfaction in the Lord, you will be transformed.

Many people tell me they are afraid to legalize food. They think that they might choose to eat sugar all day long. Well, eating salads and vegetables and diet foods under restraint and then bingeing out of frustration is just as unhealthy. After all, feeling deprived is not healthy. Other behaviors that make you feel ashamed or frustrated are not healthy either.

It's true that eating junk food from morning to evening is not a balanced diet, but sooner or later, you will crave the healthy foods you need. And when you do, you will eat them. This is because you want them and because you have a choice. At that point, you won't be afraid to make food choices, because you really will believe you are in control. Now *that* is what is called healthy!

What Are Your Favorite Foods?

Take a few moments to think about some of your favorite foods. What five things would top your list? You know the ones . . . the ones you wish had zero calories . . . the ones that are so hard to stop consuming. These are the foods you may often try to avoid but find yourself bingeing on when you come face-to-face with them.

1.
2.
3.
4.
5.

Consider the favorite foods you wrote down. Circle the ones that really seem to take you over the edge. Leave the top three out of this exercise for a few weeks as you build your confidence. Next, choose one or two of the others to test the waters.

Let's say you chose chocolate . . . sounds good to me! The last thing you want to do is go out and buy a full pound of yummy nuts and chews! That would be silly. Instead, go to your favorite candy store at the mall and look at all the great choices. Remind yourself that you can have whatever you want. Now, just choose one or two pieces. Make sure you've had a great breakfast and lunch before you treat yourself. Drink a big glass of water and then slowly enjoy your chocolate. Imagine yourself completely satisfied. Since you can do this any time you want, you won't feel like you want to rush back in the store and buy three more pieces. Get the idea?

Now, go ahead and legalize food this week and get in touch with how you feel. Record your observations.

- What foods did you eat?
- How did you feel about legalizing them?
- Are there any foods you are afraid to legalize?
- What else did you learn?

Shelving Troublesome Foods

In the quest to overcome emotional eating, you may find that certain things have a very strong pull on you emotionally. As you work on your self-talk and build your motivational muscles, it may help to put these foods out of reach for a while.

Choose "safe" times when you feel in control to test your ability to eat a small amount of these trigger foods without going overboard. Keep working on your self-talk until you believe you are in control.

It will take time to establish total comfort in this area. First, spend time really understanding the principles taught in chapter 8, *You Are What You Think*. Each time you are faced with a food choice, consider the "Six Ds" strategy below.

Determine how important your body is compared to the food you want.

Develop new self-talk messages.

Distract yourself from the temptation.

Distance yourself from the food.

Delay eating for ten minutes when you get the "urge."

Do it . . . do it . . . do it!

—— *#2—Getting in Tune with Your Hunger*

Getting in tune with your hunger is another important element in taking control of emotional eating. Can you tell the difference between what we call physiological hunger and what we call emotional hunger? Many of us have lost touch with our natural hunger. What is hunger to you? How does it feel? Do you feel it very often?

It is important to tune in and learn to feed our true hunger with food. Our emotional or "mouth" hunger cannot always be fed every time we get a signal. It's all right to feel hunger. It may seem slightly uncomfortable, but remember, this exercise will help you get in tune with your body's actual physical need for food. No matter how much stored fat you may have, you still have a need to eat every day. So listen to your body (and your stomach) when it tells you, "It's time to eat now!"

Your stomach is only about the size of a fist, and it most comfortably holds about two to four cups of solid food at one time. If you eat more than that, it begins to overstretch to accommodate the excess volume. By consistently overfilling your stomach, it gets adjusted to being in an enlarged state. When it is not filled to overfull, you feel falsely hungry. The best way to avoid this dilemma is never to overfill it!

Some interesting studies reveal how smart our bodies are without any help from us. For example, your body knows about how many calories you usually burn at certain times during the day. If you eat more than your body can burn in a given period of time, it almost immediately stores any dietary fat you have eaten. We just can't fool our awesome machine! It knows and operates on truth. So it is important for us to get tuned in to the reality of what we are eating—and why.

I'm going to be talking about hunger on a scale from 1 to 5. An explanation of each rating follows.

The Hunger Scale

1—I'm absolutely starving! You feel like you could eat anything in sight. You're getting grouchy and shaky, and food is all you can think about!

2—I'm slightly hungry. You may feel some twinges or rumbling in your belly. It definitely feels empty, and you're thinking it's time to get some food. This is the time when food actually tastes the best. Have you ever gone out to eat when you weren't hungry and ate just because you were there? It just doesn't taste as good as when your body says it's time to eat.

3—I feel neutral. You are neutral at 3—no rumblings, yet no sense of fullness either. It's a very comfortable sensation. But this is the problem: Many of us find ourselves eating when we're in this state. Sometimes we eat because the clock says it is time, and at other times because we are receiving an emotional trigger.

4—I'm physically satisfied. Two on the hunger scale means you are physically satisfied and an "early 4" means you are just barely full. Try to stop eating somewhere between a 3 and 4. As you learn to tune in to your hunger, you will identify some new things about your eating patterns. Many of us do not realize how full we are until we get up from the table. Try to tune in earlier.

5—I'm "Thanksgiving full"! Being a 5 (absolutely starving) is one extreme. This is the other one. You've had all your favorite foods, and you are so stuffed that you need to change into something a little more comfortable. In fact, you couldn't eat another bite even if someone paid you! But two hours later, you are having a little slice of pie . . . well, it is Thanksgiving, you know!

Being 1 or a 5 on the hunger scale should be avoided at all costs. Both are dangerous to your waistline. Getting to 1 on the hunger scale means your body is screaming for sugar. Remember that blood glucose needs to remain at a consistent level for you to feel high energy. When you haven't eaten for a while and your blood glucose starts to dip, your brain's immediate need for sugar overrides all your best intentions and common sense.

No matter how much fat you have stored in your reserve tanks, your body thinks it is being starved. Think about the times you have been a 1 on the hunger scale. When you finally get close to food, how and what do you eat? Most of us will choose anything quick and concentrated in high-fat or high-sugar calories. That is because your brain is screaming, "Sugar, sugar, sugar, now!" Going to 1 on the hunger scale sets you up for failure. When you finally eat, it usually is much too fast and much too much.

Of course, 5 on the scale is equally destructive. It means you have eaten way more than your body can process. You know where unburned food goes, don't you? It goes to the exact place you wish it wouldn't. It goes to its favorite retreat on your body . . . maybe your hips, thighs, or abdomen. Or if you hit 1 frequently, your excess fat will store just about anywhere with no trouble at all!

Hunger Evaluation

Assess your hunger before and after you eat, using the following scale:

1 = Extremely hungry—feels uncomfortable

2 = Slightly hungry—not uncomfortable

3 = Neutral

4 = Beginning to get full

5 = Very full—feeling uncomfortable

1. Record what number you are on the hunger scale when you begin to eat and when you finish.
   Beginning: When finished:
2. Pay close attention to your hunger pains. How does it feel to be in physiological hunger?
3. Did you confuse "mouth hunger" with physiological hunger?

Hunger Scale Questions to Answer in Seven to Ten Days

1. Are you fine-tuning your hunger and eating what you want when you're truly hungry? □ Yes □ No
2. Do you know where the desire is coming from? Are you usually hungry when you eat? □ Yes □ No
3. What is your "average" hunger when you decide to eat?
4. Are you avoiding 1 on the hunger scale? □Yes □ No
5. Are you avoiding 5 on the hunger scale? □Yes □ No
6. If you're not really hungry when you eat, then you must be emotionally hungry. What are you really feeling?

   □ Bored

   □ Frustrated

   □ Helpless

   □ Angry

   □ Tired

   □ Happy

   □ Scared

   □ Nervous

   □ Lonely

   □ Upset

7. How many times each day are you thinking about food or popping something into your mouth when you're not even hungry? _____

Remember, you're not on a diet and there are no forbidden foods. So you can eat what you want, when you want it. It tastes and feels so much better when you are truly hungry! When you do decide to eat, think about what will really satisfy you. Is it sweet or sour? Smooth or crunchy? Spicy, salty, hot, or cold?

In order to get a handle on your eating, it is important to make sure you get both physically and psychologically satisfied when you eat. For the brain to register satisfaction, you need to engage in about fifteen to twenty minutes of eating. The key is to slow down. What is your eating environment like? Are you usually

165

doing something else while you are eating? Do you often find yourself eating standing up? Eating on the run? Slow down and fully concentrate on the eating experience. Many times, we don't even remember what our food tasted like because we've been talking, reading, or watching television. We have lost the full joy and pleasure of eating.

Naturally Thin Eating

If you've ever lived with a naturally thin person, you may have noticed some key ways they relate to food. Some commonalities include:

- They eat when they are hungry and stop when they are comfortably full.
- They eat what really appeals to them at the time, rather than whatever is convenient.
- They eat slowly and enjoy every bite.
- They forget about food until they are hungry again.

How do you develop this kind of healthy eating pattern? Self-discovery and practice, practice, practice. Record your hunger scale before and after you eat. Record some of your discoveries in a small spiral notebook you can carry with you. You can use it in a variety of ways during your initial weeks of personal evaluation. (Remember that we learn from observation, imitation, and repetition.)

—— *#3—Identifying Your Eating Triggers*

Common emotional eating triggers include depression, anxiety, boredom, loneliness, frustration, and feelings of inadequacy. Identify core issues and look for long-term solutions that will reduce or eliminate the emotions that induce nonproductive behaviors.

Answer each question as Never (N), Almost never (AN), Frequently (F), or Always (A). Then tally the frequency of your responses.

1. When I am frustrated or overwhelmed, eating can make me feel better.
2. When I am nervous or stressed, eating helps calm me down.
3. If someone criticizes me or disapproves of me, I often find myself wanting to eat.
4. Eating soothes me when I feel sad.
5. Food and eating make things even better when I am very happy.
6. Some foods I eat make me feel guilty, and then I give up and eat even more.
7. My anger is reduced when I indulge in foods I like.
8. If I get in an argument with someone special to me, I feel like eating to ease the pain.
9. I frequently eat to pass the time when I am bored.
10. When I feel inferior to someone, I eat to feel better.
11. I eat more when my life seems too busy or out of control.
12. When I am mad at myself, I eat more.
13. When everything seems to be going wrong, I eat to feel better.
14. I snack a lot while I work, drive, or do certain mundane tasks.
15. I often eat before I identify any hunger or need to eat.

Analyze your results (tally your responses).

Never: _____ Almost never: _____ Frequently: _____
Always: _____

How did you do? If you have many "Frequently" or "Always" answers, you should spend time tuning in to what is really going on. Sometimes emotional eating is as simple as the fact that you have developed some bad habits. Other times, it is an issue of unhealthy self-talk messages overriding all your best attempts. Read the answers again. What do you really believe? Rewrite those messages in a positive way and say them to yourself daily. Use your new messages to help you change your underlying belief system about your emotional relationship to food.

Journal your eating patterns. Journals have been around for centuries. They have played an important role throughout history as a means of measuring progress along a particular path. The use of a private journal is very common whenever people have a fixed goal or are having difficulty attaining that goal. The journal becomes a self-testing place for personal reflection and "inner conversations."

Almost everyone at one time has eaten in response to some kind of emotional arousal. If you desire to reduce the frequency of your emotional eating occurrences, you must identify your "eating triggers." A journal will help you keep a record of your behavior and evaluate any common threads. In order to evaluate your eating patterns effectively, it is recommended that you journal your emotional eating for at least seven days.

A typical food diary has an entry for every time something is eaten. It may include:

- the time of day
- the time spent eating
- the place where eating took place
- any other activities done while eating
- your mood at the time of eating
- the food and amount eaten
- the level of hunger at the time
- an estimate of the number of calories or other nutritional information on the food eaten

Once you identify your patterns, it's time to decide what you are going to do about it. Do it now! Many of us tend to procrastinate and wait until the perfect time to start new habits or implement change. There really is no perfect time. Chances are you will always be busy. You will always have challenges or other priorities tugging at you. So each day, ask yourself, "How important is my body and my health to me?" If it is important, and it should be, do something about it. It doesn't have to take a lot of time. It doesn't have to be a perfect effort. Just small steps, day after day after day.

Remember that you believe what you tell yourself most often. If you want to feel in control of your food choices, you must tell yourself that you are . . . again and again and again. As you work "beneath the surface" on taking control of your food choices and eating patterns, use some of the techniques I'll share in the next few chapters to help you balance your energy equation without dieting.

— The Positive Cycle

One of the most important principles I've learned in overcoming emotional eating is that I always do much better when I'm well rested and my energy level is high. Practice the "Nutrition for Maximum Energy" principles (NutriMax Six) I will teach you in chapter 12. Establish a strong base with a nutritious breakfast and lunch every day. You will be amazed at how many of your cravings diminish.

Your increased energy will prompt you to become more active. Your activity will further increase your energy and decrease your appetite. Just taking better care of yourself will give you a sense of well-being that can have a dramatic impact on many of your choices and habits. Soon this positive cycle will dominate your life!

As a recovered compulsive eater and bulimic, I know how painful and frustrating emotional eating can be. Please believe me when I say that there is hope! Don't condemn yourself when you succumb to old patterns. Work on changing your perspective and cutting your losses.

In years past, I would willfully determine to control my cravings for sweets or junk food. If I finally gave in and had one chocolate chip cookie, it tasted so good that I would have another two or three. After three, I felt so guilty that I ate a dozen more just because I had blown it! The damage didn't come from three or even four cookies. The damage came when I caved in and ate the whole box. And after the first three, they didn't even taste very good.

It took time for me to change those old thinking patterns. It took time to believe I could be in control. Today I can eat a little more than I should and then stop and say, "Hey, that tasted great! Now I'll just have to burn a few more calories and eat lighter at dinner!" You know what? It works! Today, I know I am in control of my food choices. I also know you are in control of yours. Soon, you will know it too!

— 11
——— **burning fat**
— **to the max**

— The Obesity Epidemic

Despite the fitness craze, fat-free foods, artificial sweeteners, and supposed "fat-burning nutrients," Americans are getting fatter and fatter. Recent statistics indicate that almost 80 percent of Americans are heavier than they should be for good health. Burning fat is no longer primarily a cosmetic issue—obesity has become a national epidemic. And children are gaining weight at an alarming rate as well. In fact, experts agree that obesity has become one of the primary causes of many diseases and premature deaths, second only to smoking. Sadly, both are within our control.

Whether you're carrying a lot of excess fat or just a little, it is important to learn how to keep your fat stores in check. As I've already said, our bodies are functioning in the same way they were thousands of years ago. And way back then, very few people had weight problems. So if our bodies didn't change, what did? Our lifestyles and our habits! Over the last decade I've been asked over and over, "Will your program work for me?" For many years, I would state confidently, "Yes!" That's because I know the principles I teach are based on truth—truth about how God designed our bodies, minds, and spirits. However, programs and principles don't create change unless you act on them. And it is equally important to apply these truths appropriately. Sometimes in our zeal to change, we go too far. That was the case with my client "Kelly."

— A Wrong Lifestyle Choice

Have you ever run into someone and hardly recognized her because she'd lost so much weight? The transformation is incredible, and you are thrilled for her. The first question you ask is, "How did you do it?" Perhaps she tells you it was a liquid diet. You wonder, *How will she keep it off?* After all, she can't live on liquids forever. Will her lean new body be enough to keep her motivated enough to do the right things?

Sadly, this is rarely the case. More often than not, the next time you see her, she will be back to her "old" self. Why? Because to lose weight permanently, you have to get it off the same way you're going to keep it off. I've said that hundreds of times over the past ten years.

Kelly had struggled with her weight all her life. At barely 5 feet tall, her small frame strained under her 225-pound weight. She came to me in desperation and joined one of my lifestyle classes at a local women's fitness club. She soaked up all the information and truths about how the body burns fat and began implementing many new lifestyle changes immediately.

Most people who have struggled with excessive weight for many years have been on dozens of diets. They are good at restricting food using that all-or-nothing approach I've talked about. So I encouraged Kelly not to go on another diet. We identified several ways she could modify how she ate without feeling deprived. She assured me she was eating well and was committed to burning more calories than she ate every day. She felt liberated that by increasing her activity, she could eat a reasonable amount of food and still lose weight.

Over many months, Kelly began to shed considerable weight. When I caught up with her a year later, she was a shadow of her former self. She had lost over one hundred pounds! What I didn't know was she had made one lifestyle change in the process that would be her undoing.

While the concept of increasing her calorie burn by moving more was a healthy one, I had no idea she had taken it to an extreme. Kelly had been exercising two to three hours a day almost every day of the week for the past year. I cautioned her with a stern warning. "Kelly, do you really believe you can keep up this level of activity for the rest of your life? You may not always have the time. You may not always even want to spend that much time in the gym. And more importantly, even though you are much leaner, you're likely to get injured." It was a miracle she hadn't injured herself . . . yet!

Six months later, when I ran into Kelly at a local restaurant, she had gained forty pounds. A foot injury had prevented her from working out for several months. A year later, her weight had crept up seventy-five pounds. Once her foot was healed, she had lost the motivation to go back to her old regime. The next time I saw her at the mall, she saw me from a distance and clearly wanted to avoid me. I pretended not to see her although she was hard to miss—she was larger than when we'd first met. My heart broke. What had gone wrong?

Kelly had made a lifestyle change she couldn't maintain most days for the rest of her life. By exercising two or more hours a day, her calorie burn exceeded 1,200 calories a day in activity alone. Combined with her resting metabolic rate (how many calories one burns at rest alone), she was burning over 2,500 calories a day. Kelly had been able to eat 2,500 calories a day and stay lean . . . as long as she burned those extra 1,200 calories each day. When she got injured, all activity ceased. However, she kept eating the same. And the weight piled on. She hadn't made a reasonable lifestyle change she could live with. It is essential that you make changes you can maintain—not perfectly, but more often than not. Was there something wrong with the truths I'd taught Kelly? No, there was something wrong with the way she applied them. Don't replace one addiction for another. Overindulgence on exercise does not glorify God more than overeating, just because you look better. Juggling the balls of life requires a balance of priorities, an accurate perspective, and proper application of truth.

With that in mind, please take the simple principles I will teach you in the next pages and make reasonable changes to your lifestyle. My goal is for you to understand exactly how your body burns and stores the three fuel sources: carbohydrates, proteins, and fats. Once you understand this, you will be able to make wise decisions and discern why so many diets and diet products are more hype than help.

— Throw Out Your Scale

Before we focus on the key fat-burning factors, I'd like to address the issue of your bathroom scale. Your first assignment is: Throw it out! You may be wondering, "A book called *Scale Down* is telling me to get rid of my scale?" Yes, that's exactly right . . . put your *scale down!* It gives you very limited information.

Has this ever happened to you? You're sticking to your diet, attempting to lose those extra pounds, and trying to get more exercise or activity into your life. You need a little encouragement and want to know how well you're doing, so you jump on the scale. You know you've been doing the right things, but the scale says you weigh more, even though you had to cinch up your belt a notch. How frustrating! So you just give up and go back to your old ways.

As I described in chapter 4, you can only lose about one pound of fat every two days if you absolutely starve yourself. Yet since our body is 65 to 75 percent water, our water weight can shift 2–3 pounds a day with very little effort. How can you know what has really happened by weighing every day? You can't!

I'm a good example of someone who used the scale and failed. In my early twenties, I did all sorts of unhealthy things to lose weight. I would get on the scale almost every single morning. One year after taking diet pills for a few months, I dropped from 150 to 120 pounds and from a size 14 to a size 9. I was thrilled! I assumed I had lost lots of fat. Sadly, within six months my weight was creeping right back up, and I looked fatter than before!

Today, at 50 years old, I stay about a size 6 . . . and I weigh about 138 pounds! That's 18 pounds more than when I had lost 30 pounds and was a size 9 after diet pills! What's the difference? It's the difference between muscle and fat. Muscle weighs more. So let go of the numbers and throw out your scale!

If you do the right things, your best body will follow. Who cares what the numbers say? If you want an accurate assessment of how your body is changing, use a tape measure and record your measurements every few months. Or pick a pair of tight jeans and put them on every few weeks. When they fit comfortably, you can really celebrate your progress. And the best measure of all—stand in front of the mirror!

— Burning Fat . . . The "One Thing"

I've said it before, and I'll keep on saying it: From a purely physical standpoint, the most important fat-burning factor is, was, and always will be—calories in versus calories out. Everything else is secondary. I encourage you to stop researching every new diet, supplement, and designer food that you encounter. Just focus on those two key things every day, and you will have fat-burning success.

You can take fat-burning supplements, follow special food-combining diets, and eat low-fat or high-protein diets until you're blue in the face. But the only time actual fat loss occurs is when the body burns more calories than it takes in. That's it. Every pound of fat lost on every diet is due to one thing—burning more calories than you consume.

—— *The Bottom Line to Your Bottom Line*

It is true that genetics, health, and diet history influence a person's ability to burn fat effectively. We don't all burn at the same rate. However, the same principles of fat metabolism hold true. It sometimes takes longer and is harder for some people to get results; often those who struggle the most are the very ones who have damaged their natural ability to burn fat because of chronic dieting. But if we follow some basic principles, we can all move in a positive direction, despite our past choices. Many health experts agree that only about 30 percent of our health (including weight) is impacted by things out of our control. Fortunately, about 70 percent is directly within our own power of choice.

The body is a calorie-burning and storing machine. We eat food, and our body either uses it for fuel or stores it. When people lose fat, they are using their fat storage as fuel. And there's only one time our body will use already stored fat for fuel—when we burn more calories than we eat. It all comes down to calories in versus calories out. That's what I call the energy equation.

We've already discovered that by eating an extra five calories per day, we will store an excess twenty pounds of fat over thirty years! It doesn't take much to become an American statistic. However, the biggest reason we are getting fatter is not simply from eating more. We are also moving far less. We think that our lives are normal, but they're not. Most of us lead a very sedentary existence.

In order to manage your fat effectively, it's important to work on both sides of the energy equation—both the "in" and the "out." Most people focus primarily on changing the "in" side of the equation (what they're eating) when they want to lose weight. That's why so many people go on diets. The truth is, most of us underestimate how much we are really eating. But that's only half the story.

Burning calories is the other side of the equation. Let's recap what we learned earlier. The average American woman only burns about 1,700 calories each day. However, in the early 1900s, most people burned at least 25 percent more calories. Why? Think about how they lived. There were no power vacuums or automatic washers, no drive-through restaurants or dry cleaners. People walked everywhere and engaged in physical labor every day. Now just imagine your life. For many of us, the extent of our exercise includes getting into the shower and walking to our cars. We drive to undercover parking, take elevators to our offices, roll around on wheeled chairs, and e-mail our business associates.

So while it's important to bring nutrition and eating habits in line, lack of activity is an equally important issue. To get and stay lean for life, we must make a lifestyle change that includes increased daily activity. In our fast-paced, low-activity society, most of us will need to purposely add activity into our lives.

There are 3,500 calories in one pound of fat. Visualize one pound of fat as a pound of raw hamburger on your body. It's really quite sizeable! If you eat enough calories and actively burn 500 calories more than you eat each day, you will burn off about one pound of fat every week. That could be 52 pounds in one year! And you won't have to change your life dramatically. As I've said many times before, small, consistent changes in your behavior add up in a big way over time.

—— *Do the Math and Get Moving!*

A general rule of thumb is for every 100 extra calories burned per day, you will lose about one pound of fat per month. For a 140-pound woman, that is the equivalent of walking about one mile. So 200 extra calories equals approximately 20 pounds in one year; 400 equals 40; 500 equals 50, and so forth. Of course, this is assuming your caloric intake does not go up! Sounds pretty simple, doesn't it? It is! Our greatest obstacle is discipline and consistency.

Don't get frustrated and try to get that excess weight off too quickly. A month or two down the road, you'll feel exhausted and irritable. That is not a lifestyle change. It's an all-or-nothing approach, and it rarely works.

—— *Do the Math and Decrease Your Input*

If you want to make a little faster progress, take a look at the food you're eating. Decreasing the calories in your diet could save you one hundred to three hundred calories per day. Just eliminate some of your fun foods or "empty" carbohydrates like French bread, crackers, and bagels that you thought were safe because they are fat free. It's pretty easy to find small ways to reduce your caloric intake by two hundred to three hundred calories a day. (I'll give you many more ideas in the next chapter.)

To lose that twenty pounds in six months, all you have to do is increase your activity (or calorie burn) by two hundred calories a day and decrease your caloric intake two hundred calories per day. The key to losing fat permanently is to make changes you can live with. This is not about fast . . . it's about permanent and painless.

— Your Body's Three Fuel Sources

I want you to think about your refrigerator for a moment. If you were facing a long, cold winter, you'd stock it with a good supply of food in order to be prepared. Your body is a refrigerator of sorts. It stores three types of fuel: carbohydrates, proteins, and fats. The body maintains a very delicate balance when it comes to fuel. Second only to oxygen, it needs a constant

178

source of glucose; the brain must have a steady supply of glucose, or sugar, in order to function. Glucose is generated from the body's number one fuel source: carbohydrates. Yet look at all the high-protein, low-carbohydrate diets that are so popular. Let me explain why this is such a big mistake.

—— *Fuel Source #1—Carbohydrates*

The brain receives this fuel source in the form of blood sugar. When our blood sugar drops too low, we become irritable, shaky, or even faint. However, overfilling our bodies with too many simple carbohydrates (or sugar) is a problem as well. The pancreas, which produces insulin, must make sure we don't have too much sugar circulating in the bloodstream. If we do, it goes to work in short order to get that extra sugar out of the blood and ultimately stored in a fat cell. Overeating sugar and refined carbohydrates is a primary factor in developing adult-onset diabetes.

A 140-pound person has approximately 200 calories of glucose circulating in the bloodstream at all times. There's also about 2,000 carbohydrate calories in the form of glycogen stored in the muscles and liver. Under normal circumstances the blood sugar is maintained by accessing these glycogen stores. In addition to glycogen, we have two other fuel sources available in storage: proteins and fats.

At rest or during very moderate activity like sitting or standing, our bodies only use about 5 to 10 percent of fat for fuel. The fuel we do use during these low activity moments is 90 to 95 percent carbohydrate. When we restrict our calories by dieting but don't exercise, the first thing our bodies use is our glycogen, which is found in our muscles and liver. That's because it's a readily accessible form of carbohydrate, our bodies' favorite fuel.

When we first start a diet, the reason we seem to lose weight so fast is because as the body uses up glycogen, it releases relatively large amounts of water. The drop on the scale is mostly water and not fat! But what do you really want to lose? You want to lose the extra and unnecessary fat. In addition, our bodies actually burn fat best in the flame of carbohydrate (when some dietary carbohydrate is present). So when our carbohydrate stores are depleted, fat metabolism is actually compromised.

Fuel Source #2—Proteins

Our dietary proteins (or amino acids) are used to replace or build muscles and organs in our body. Proteins are also used for most of our transport systems, such as hormones, enzymes, neurotransmitters, and immune system elements. But most people don't realize that these essential systems are often the first compromised when we fail to nourish our bodies properly.

Once the glycogen stores are low, we may feel irritable or lethargic because our blood sugar is not well supported. Our bodies now go in search of another fuel source to support the blood sugar. Often, stored protein is easier to access than the fat. Now we're really in trouble. When we restrict calories, we sacrifice protein for energy instead of burning fat. We haven't lost any significant fat, our lean body mass is decreasing, and our metabolism is starting to drop.

Fuel Source #3—Fats

Fat is like high-octane fuel. It has nine calories per gram, while carbohydrates and proteins have only four. It's usually the first fuel to be stored if we eat more than we are burning, and it is often the last to be burned. However, with sustained activity (most specifically aerobic activity), it becomes a primary source of fuel.

It's not just the fat in our diets that is making us fat. After all, if you burn all the calories you eat, you won't store anything. And if you eat no fat but still consume more carbohydrate or protein calories than you burn, the excess calories will be stored as fat. Eating too much fat is obviously a problem from both a health and fat management standpoint. However, cutting down on fat alone is not the answer. Those of us who love food tend to over-compensate and eat more carbohydrates. Ultimately our total caloric intake stabilizes or even increases. The answer is to get a balance of all three macronutrients. A healthy range of fat is between 15 to 25 percent of our total calories, with most of those coming from healthy sources such as flaxseed, canola oil, or olive oil. I'll give you many specific nutritional recommendations in the next chapter.

After a short trip through the liver, unused fatty acids hook up with proteins and get transported to adipose tissue. There they sit and wait to be called out as future fuel sources. And as you've already heard, stored fat is only called out when we are burning more calories than we are eating. Otherwise, they're like money in our savings account, just waiting to be transferred to checking!

—— *Survival of the Fattest*

The adult human has a set number of fat cells, which enlarge to accommodate fat storage. Fat cells are formed at specific times of growth, such as infancy, adolescence, and during pregnancy. So later in life when we work to lose or gain weight, we are just shrinking or expanding our existing cells. These cells are in a constant state of metabolism.

Our body is the most intricate and complex machine ever designed. It is programmed to protect you in every way possible, no matter what you do, and it cares more about your well-being and survival than about how thin you are. Your body doesn't give a hoot what our society says the standard should be. It isn't a bit worried about that cellulite on your thighs or your expanding waistline. In fact, it's probably quite happy because a nice storage of reserve fuel is available in case of famine (or a self-imposed starvation diet).

— Five Fat-Burning Factors

Boosting and sustaining a strong metabolism is influenced by many physiological factors. Two are out of your control—gender and genetics. The rest are up to you! The five fat-burning factors are:

1. Gender
2. Genetics
3. Exercise/activity
4. Nutrition
5. Muscle maintenance

Let's take a closer look at each one.

—— *Factor #1—Gender*

God delivered you with a blueprint stamped male or female. That's just the way it is; we may as well celebrate it. And the inherent differences in men and women influence our fat-burning and storing capabilities.

Women were designed for a specific purpose. From a purely physical standpoint, our bodies were first and foremost designed to support another life. This is not a comment to spur a philosophical debate. It's a fact. Our gender has a direct influence on our hormones, which tell all our related body systems just how prepared we are for that specific mission, desired or not. From puberty on, our internal chemistry is working based on this presumption, month after month after month.

The hormones involved in this process stimulate our fat cells to work like mighty soldiers to ensure we never run short of fuel. The female body wants to know that it's capable to carry or nur-

182

ture an infant. That's why some adolescent girls take so long to begin menstruation. If their body-fat percentage is too low, their body is not in a position to support a child, so they don't ovulate. In the same way, when women become too lean through too much exercise, stress, or dieting, their periods may stop. What an incredible machine!

If you think about it, the female body must be an excellent fat-storing machine to ensure the perpetuation of life. If you store fat well, your body is doing a great job. Now, that doesn't mean we want to store too much extra fat, but it is a natural and healthy process when not taken to the extreme. And that is why it generally is more difficult for women to have the body our culture promotes.

Our specific gender affects the two key enzymes that play a role in fat metabolism. They include the lipogenic enzymes that help us store fat, and the lipolytic enzymes that help us burn fat. Lipogenic and lipolytic . . . which ones do you think women have more of? You've got it—the lipogenic, fat-storing enzymes. Darn! One of the reasons men burn fat more readily than women is because the lipolytic fat-burning enzymes are activated in the mitochondria of muscle cells, and men have more muscle mass than women.

Have you ever noticed that when a man decides to work on the old love handles or drop a few pounds, all he has to do is cut down a little on calories or just notch up his exercise? It doesn't seem fair, but that's the way it is. In our action plan, I'll give you some ideas to stimulate muscle growth and lipolytic fat-burning enzyme activity.

Factor #2—Genetics

Our genetic blueprint is predetermined before we're even born. If your directions read "Stop growing at five foot two," nothing you can do will make you five foot seven. Similarly, if your blueprint reads "long arms" or "short legs" or "a gymnast's body" or "a fashion model's body" . . . that's the way it is. So there are a few things we need to accept and celebrate. The good news is that we have incredible influence in making our specific body type its very best!

I speak with many women who are frustrated because they work so hard on their nutrition and exercise programs and still see fat on their bodies. The reality is they may always see some fat in natural areas like the hips, buttocks, or thighs. How much will depend on the fat-fighting factors within their control. Keep in mind that your body will respond best to moderate and consistent change. You have control over what you eat and how much you move, and these choices and behaviors will influence how you burn fat much more significantly than gender or genetics.

─── *Factor #3—Exercise/Activity*

The easiest way to burn off those adipose stores is to move, move, move! When we engage in large muscle, sustained activity such as walking, biking, swimming, or even dancing, we significantly increase the amount of fat being burned for fuel. These types of activities are considered aerobic because we're able to sustain them for long periods of time without running out of sufficient oxygen.

When we are at rest or are moving sporadically, the caloric demands on our bodies are minimal. An average-sized woman burns about one to two calories per minute; a man about two to four. In a resting or moderately sedentary state, it's easy for the body to convert glycogen into glucose at a sufficient rate. But when the body starts to move aerobically, it gets a little concerned that it may run out of glycogen, its preferred fuel source.

To conserve glycogen, the body tells the fat cells to start releasing their stored fuel; now the body is ready to sustain aerobic activity. The percentage of fat burned begins to increase steadily from about 5 percent to over 50 percent in the first thirty minutes of aerobic activity, and this will continue throughout the aerobic workout. It's easy to see the most efficient and healthy way to access stored body fat is through frequent aerobic exercise, especially at intervals of thirty minutes or more.

Just imagine farmers at the turn of the century stopping in the middle of the field to check if their heart rate was in their "target zone"! This concept of exercising in a zone at least three times a week is only necessary because our lives are so sedentary. Most of us can't quit our jobs and go back to growing our own food. And we probably can't give up our cars for walking or riding horses.

Therefore, we do need to make a conscious effort to get our bodies moving. For some, that means exercise. From my perspective, the "E" word represents a very specific activity designed to work the body for an intended result. It has its advantages. Exercise tends to be time efficient and, if done properly, can be very effective.

Additionally, you can choose to adopt a more active lifestyle in general. Parking farther from the store, taking stairs, walking your dog, dancing, or working in the yard are examples of lifestyle activities that can make a big difference in your overall health and calorie burn.

In this day and age, the ideal is a combination of both. You have to decide on both your fitness and weight-management goals. If you want to be a more efficient calorie burner, you'll want to improve your fitness level. Then you can move at a higher intensity and burn calories more effectively. Walking a mile or running a mile burns about the same number of calories. The runner just gets finished faster!

Aerobic exercise is key. Let's make sure you've got this very important point. To access significant stored fat and protect your metabolism, you must move aerobically. So what happens if you eat less than you burn but don't get aerobic exercise?

We have to use up some form of stored fuel when we eat less than we burn. But without the stimulus of exercise, the body usually will go to the glycogen stores first; only small amounts of stored fat will be used for energy. And should the body run short on glycogen, it may begin to use muscle. Using one pound of muscle for energy will only supply the body with 600 calories of fuel, whereas a pound of fat supplies 3,500 calories of fuel. Yes, you will lose a pound of weight on the scale, but it won't be fat, and your metabolism will drop in the process. A pound of fat only burns about three calories per day. A pound of muscle burns about fifty! Losing a pound of muscle could decrease your metabolism enough to *gain* a pound of fat in one year.

So remember, fat metabolism is only maximized when you move your body aerobically. During this activity, calorie burn increases dramatically from one to two calories per minute to five to fifteen per minute, depending on your size and the intensity of the exercise. Maximum fat metabolism occurs at about thirty minutes of sustained movement.

Understanding how your body stores and burns food motivates you to make the right choices. I love to imagine my body gobbling up all those fat molecules from my thighs every time I go for a walk or a run. And I am sure my thighs would be much larger if I didn't get my aerobic activity at least six times each week.

I hope these facts will help you appreciate how important exercise is to getting and staying lean. Make it a lifestyle! (Refer to chapter 14 for specific exercise and fitness recommendations.)

——— *Factor #4—Nutrition*

With all this talk about burning calories, you wouldn't think that undereating is a problem, but it is. Low-calorie eating will damage your metabolism. Even 1,200 calories is too low for most people.

We each burn a large number of calories while just resting. Lying still for twenty-four hours, you burn about 60 to 70 percent of your total calories. That rate of calorie burn is called your resting metabolic rate, or RMR. It is different for everyone, and it's determined largely by your age, weight, and lean body mass (or muscle). It can also be influenced by other genetic or hormonal factors. To protect and enhance your metabolism, never eat less than your RMR for a sustained period of time. Otherwise, after several days, your body's engine will begin to gradually slow down.

Perhaps my relationship with my car will help you better understand how this works. Have you ever waited to fill up your gas tank until after the warning light goes on? I bet you have! I do it all the time. In fact, I've gone so far as to figure out that I have exactly twenty-five miles after my light goes on before I actually run out of gas. You would think my car would figure this out and start to conserve fuel when I get that close to the bottom of the tank. Nope! It just keeps burning gas at the same number of miles per gallon.

However, the body is a much smarter machine. What happens when you consistently eat less calories than your resting metabolic rate requires is that your body starts to have a conversation with itself that sounds something like this:

"Hey, here she goes again. She's not even going to feed us enough calories for basic survival. Slow the engines . . . all systems cool down to basic maintenance. We will not starve!"

Yes, your body actually slows down the rate at which you burn calories. So for many dieters, a dangerous cycle begins. And over time, your Ferrari engine has been converted to an incredible economy car—like the original Volkswagen Bug! Now this is great if you're worried about never having enough food on the table or going into a time of severe famine. But for those of us who enjoy food, it's best to keep those engines burning high.

187

As a 50-year-old, 5 foot 7 inch, 138-pound female, my resting metabolic rate is about 1,400 calories per day. Yet how many of us have been on 800-, 1,000-, or 1,200-calorie diets? For a ballpark idea of your RMR, multiply your current weight times 10 for women and 11 for men. If you are 150 pounds, your resting rate is about 1,500 calories.

New studies have shown that even moderate dieting creates a rebound phenomenon. This means that the body wants to bounce back to its old weight. Only slow and steady weight loss that doesn't "shock" your body will last.

Eat and Burn All Day Long

Once fat is stored, our bodies are resistant to letting it go. The best solution is to avoid overeating. The overall objective is to balance the intake of protein, carbohydrates, and fat in percentages optimal to fuel the body. It is equally important to ensure we burn all the calories we eat by maintaining an active lifestyle.

How does the body store fat throughout the day? Unfortunately, it doesn't wait until the end of a twenty-four-hour period, check the balance sheet of calories in versus calories out, and decide how many grams of fat to bank in the reserve tank. Instead, it goes through this process all day long. Once again, imagine that your body is like a car. When you go to the gas station to fuel up, you can only put in as much fuel as the tank will hold. If your tank is sixteen gallons, the gasoline will spill onto your shoes if you try to overfill it! Oh, if only our bodies operated the same way! But our incredible machine would never waste an ounce of fuel. We have almost unlimited storage tanks—fat cells.

Let's review. Our bodies will store excess calories in the form of glycogen, protein, or fat until they are needed for energy. If we eat more calories than we burn, very little stored fat will be utilized. If we burn more calories than we eat, we will access stored calories.

Our bodies process limited amounts of calories each time we eat. If we can't use all the calories within a short period of time, we store them as fat. The solution is to eat several small meals or substantial snacks throughout the day. Start early with breakfast and then eat and burn, eat and burn all day long.

If your body were a car with a five-gallon tank, five gallons would be the maximum you could fuel up at one time. You'd be forced to burn fuel before you could take on more. Consider your body just that way and imagine that each gallon represents about one hundred calories. That means you could only take in about five hundred calories at one time without spilling over into the reserve tanks. Of course, larger women and men might have larger six, seven, or eight-gallon tanks, but the principle is the same.

That is, our bodies process calories best when we eat approximately what we will need over a three- to four-hour time period. In fact, some interesting studies indicate that our bodies may be so tuned in to our needs that they almost immediately begin storing fat if we overfill our tanks at any one time. For example, if you generally burn about five hundred calories between 6:00 A.M. and 10:00 A.M., your body will notice if you eat more than your usual five hundred calories. Your body knows these calories will not be used immediately, so like an incredibly efficient assistant, it will store them away in your fat cells until you really need them.

How do we avoid this excellent fat-storing process? Simply don't overfuel at any one time. All through the day, eat and burn, eat and burn, as if you had a maximum capacity, like your car. For women, a general rule of thumb would be about 300 to 500 calories every 4 to 5 waking hours. That would average 1,600 to 2,000 calories per day. Of course, this can vary dramatically with your personal resting metabolic rate and activity level.

All dietary calories must be digested and held in reserve for future use. The less fat we store, the less we will need to burn off later. By regulating the percentage of fat at each meal and limiting unnecessary calories, we can avoid storing too much. One thing I'd like to emphasize is the importance of breakfast. If you get in your car and leave for work in the morning, you're not going to get very far if the tank is almost empty. Most of us burn one to two calories per minute just sleeping. Our bodies need an immediate source of fuel in the morning to get going. In fact, studies show that breakfast can enhance metabolism by up to 10 percent.

Start your day right with a decent breakfast that includes protein, carbohydrates, and a good source of fiber to stabilize your blood sugar. Fat actually burns best in the "flame" of carbohydrates. We burn most of our calories in the first twelve hours of the day, but most Americans eat 50 to 60 percent of their calories after 6:00 P.M.! It just doesn't make sense to fuel up for bedtime. Just imagine all those little fat cells storing away for a long nap with you. Start to lighten up the evening meal and push those calories into the earlier part of your day.

Burn to Meet Your Natural Appestat

You can set your thermostat at home to maintain a certain level of heat. Our bodies also seem to have a pre-set "appestat"— that is, a natural inclination to eat a certain volume of food to meet our dietary requirements.

I realized some interesting things about my own personal activity and natural appestat. My resting metabolic rate is about 1,400 calories. If I don't engage in purposeful activity or exercise, I only burn about 250 to 300 active calories per day. That means on a sedentary day, I burn about 1,650 calories. However, my appestat or natural desire for food seems to consistently hover at about 2,000 calories. So if I purposely burn an extra 500 calories each day in aerobic exercise, my total calorie burn for the day is about 2,200. When I eat and burn like this, I am never hungry, I stay lean, and my body is more energized.

That may sound like a fair amount of calories for women, but it's not. Most women need approximately two thousand quality calories each day just to get enough nutrients to maintain optimal health. It seems that we're born to crave the number of calories we are designed to consume. Unfortunately, our appetite for exercise doesn't seem to follow. The problem is that we don't burn two thousand or more calories per day as we did in years past. The solution is not to eat less but to exercise more.

In addition, bad habits and out-of-control emotional eating can push our natural appestat into an unnatural appetite for more calories than we can burn. If that is your challenge, spend more time working on the principles in Chapter 10.

—— *Factor #5—Muscle Maintenance*

Toned and strengthened muscles are very hungry and burn lots of calories. One pound of fat only burns about three calories per day at rest. One pound of muscle burns up to fifty calories each day. Muscle is also more efficient in creating and releasing the lipolytic, fat-burning enzymes.

Increase the production and efficiency of your fat-burning enzymes by engaging in regular muscular conditioning exercises. A conditioned individual is much more efficient at fat burning, even at rest! There's a reward to any type of exercise called the "after burn." Those are the additional calories you burn after exercise is stopped, just because you have stimulated your metabolism. You may notice that you are warmer, which is the result of improved circulation and the fact that your muscles are burning more calories.

By doing some weight training several times each week, you can significantly improve your metabolism while you strengthen and tone your muscles. Even a ten-minute muscle workout can make a big difference if you do it with consistency. So get going and rev up your metabolic engines!

— From Knowledge to Action in Four Steps

Now that you have a clear understanding about how your body works and why it is essential to give it what it needs, it's time to put this knowledge into action. I will give you four action steps to help you balance your energy equation in the right direction. In designing your personal recipe for success, pick one or two steps at a time. Work on them until they become habits, and then add another step.

—— *Step 1—Determine Your RMR and Eat to Burn*

As you learned earlier, your body burns a certain number of calories each day just surviving. This means you need to fuel it with at least that many calories, especially since your metabolism is compromised when you eat too little. To ensure you don't slow down your engines, eat at least enough calories each day to satisfy your resting metabolic rate. Calculate your approximate RMR below.

What's Your RMR?

Women:
Weight _____ x 10 = _____
Men:
Weight _____ x 11 = _____

Does your RMR seem high to you? It may, but don't fall into old diet habits and eat less than that number. Remember that the only way to burn fat and protect your metabolism is to eat and burn. That means eat your RMR and move, move, move!

Note: If you are more than 30 percent over your recommended weight, it may seem like eating your RMR calories is excessive. In this instance, you may be able to eat slightly lower than your RMR without damaging your metabolism. If you are 50 or more

192

pounds overweight, I encourage you to seek the advice of a registered dietician or licensed professional to determine the right minimum caloric requirement for you. Our nutritional consultant, Patti Milligan, R.D., M.S., believes that most obese individuals can safely lose weight eating no more than 2,000 to 2,400 calories per day.[1]

For example, if you are a 5 foot 8 inch woman weighing 220 pounds, your RMR is about 2,200 calories. Nevertheless, it is probably safe for you to eat about 2,000 calories a day, which is 200 calories less than your RMR.

—— *Step 2—Get a Reality Check*

In a perfect world, we would crave only healthy food, eat only when we were hungry, and move all day long. Since that doesn't seem to come naturally to many of us, we have to make conscious choices to balance out our imperfect lifestyles and habits. It's time to get a reality check so that we can make those choices based on truth.

You make deposits into your calorie bank account every day in the form of food and drink. You also make withdrawals in the form of energy or calories burned. Unlike with our financial bank account, most of us would prefer to be a little overdrawn in the calorie department, burning more calories than we eat, at least until we used up all of our excess fat.

When I realized that the bottom line to fat management was calories, this simplified things for me. I felt as if I were freed up to eat the way I wanted, without so many rules. When it came to making choices about what I was going to put into my mouth, things were simple. I accepted the fact that I couldn't eat more than I burned and still have a lean body.

The advantage of understanding calories is that it gives you complete freedom to design your eating based on your personal likes and dislikes. It gives you flexibility to make midcourse corrections each day or week. It provides you with an understanding of how your body is using the fuel you're putting in. "But counting calories makes me feel like I'm dieting!" you may say. Go back to the money or checkbook example and think of calorie counting as if you were learning to manage money for the first time. At first it's easier just to spend and never budget or record. But after a few months of bouncing checks, running out of cash before you pay your bills, and paying extra fees, you soon decide it's time to get serious.

Counting calories is a temporary reality check that will give you knowledge and control of your choices. Even when you stop actively counting, you will be amazed at how the new information you've learned impacts your choices.

If you are truly serious about getting lean, it's time to bite the bullet and do a forty-day reality check. Determine what you are currently burning as well as what you are currently eating. Keep as accurate a log as possible for forty days. I know it sounds like awful drudgery. However, few of us would consider going through a whole month without deducting the checks we wrote from our check register. We know we could easily become overdrawn in our bank accounts. But that's what we do every day with our calories. If calories are the bottom line, it makes sense to know what the bottom line really is.

Note: I use an activity monitor called a Caltrac that measures both my movement calories as well as my resting metabolic rate. I have found it to be a very helpful tool for most people. You can also refer to the activity charts at the end of this chapter and estimate your daily burn based on your usual activities. The numbers are based on a 130-pound woman and a 180-pound man. Keep in mind that the number of calories you burn depends on your weight, muscle mass, and metabolism, as well as the intensity of your workout. In general, a moderate workout of any kind will burn 4 to 5 calories per minute. A highly fit person who really cranks up the intensity can burn 10 to 12 calories per minute.

——— *Step 3—Design a Calorie Budget*

You already have learned the importance of eating no fewer calories than is required for your resting metabolic rate. However, you can certainly eat more than that and still lose excess body fat.

Once you know your RMR and have a better handle on the calories you've been eating and burning, create your actual calorie budget. That means you should decide how many calories you want to consume each day and exactly what choices you will make. If you get a little off track, just make midday (or even midweek) adjustments to keep your energy equation balanced.

Experiment with the amount of activity and calorie intake that works best for you most days. I feel satisfied and in control when I can eat about 2,000 calories a day. When I eat less, I often feel deprived or hungry. With an RMR of 1,400, I need to burn about 600 active calories a day to balance my energy equation and not gain excess fat.

It took me a while to figure out the best equation to suit my lifestyle. Once I did, I experienced incredible freedom and satisfaction with my daily diet and my body. Give it a little time and experiment with the best formula for your energy equation. It will be well worth the investment!

It's all about choice. When I visit my favorite coffee shop and learn that the cinnamon roll is 600 calories, I think twice about ordering it. Is it worth a five-mile walk? Maybe . . . maybe not. My latte costs me $3.00 and 190 calories. Is it worth 20 minutes of aerobic exercise? Absolutely! I love the taste and the experience. I savor every sip.

The truth is difficult to deny. Even without counting, you will know instinctively if you are overspending your calorie budget. Life is about choices. Now you will be able to choose based on truth!

List three ways you could easily decrease your caloric intake each day.

1.
2.
3.

Note: While calories are the bottom line in fat management, they are not the only consideration when it comes to maximizing your nutrition. Blend the truths in chapter 12 with the principles in this chapter to balance maximum enjoyment with maximum health and energy. In other words, look at the whole picture.

—— *Step 4—Increase Your Burn*

Once you have determined your calorie budget, you get to choose how to spend it based on the energy equation "calories in versus calories out." So what happens if you go "over budget"? Well, you need to make a deposit by choosing to move more. Wouldn't it be nice to be able to increase your salary every time you decide to spend more money? Well, you can do just that with your calorie back account.

You're in control of the choices you make and how many extra calories you want to burn each day. List three ways you could easily increase your caloric output each day (be specific as to activity and time).

1.
2.
3.

Again, the Caltrac is an excellent tool to demonstrate accurately the exact difference between your calorie intake and your calorie output. It doesn't matter what you think you are doing. The body responds only to truth: calories in versus calories out.

If you want to lose one pound of stored body fat per week *and* maintain a healthy metabolism, here is the key:

Determine Your RMR

Eat no less than your RMR calories each day.

Burn at least 500 activity calories daily.

Lose 1 pound of body fat each week by eating 3,500 calories less than you burn (an average of 500 calories per day).

Example:

A 160-pound woman with an RMR of 1,600 eats 1,600 calories each day and burns 500 activity calories. That gives her a total 24-hour calorie burn of 2,100.

The difference is +500 calories per day.

500 calories x 7 days = 3,500 calories = 1 pound of fat

If you are at least twenty-five pounds overweight, you can safely lose two pounds per week if you are willing to burn one thousand activity calories each day. Larger individuals will burn more calories when moving, due to their larger body mass. As you get closer to your ideal weight, it will feel like dieting and deprivation to burn one thousand extra calories each day.

Remember—you are making a lifestyle change. Can you live with this new behavior most days for the rest of your life? If not . . . you probably won't keep the weight off.

— A Burning Fat Summary

I hope the truths I've shared with you thus far will help you understand the underlying physiology of your body and the psychology of your mind to move you toward leaner and healthier habits. As you've learned, it's not very complicated. We don't have to hold a Ph.D. in nutrition or exercise physiology to find the secret to lean, healthy living. It's been right under our noses all along. We simply need to get back to basics and

- eat more healthfully;
- get more active; and
- believe we can do it!

Take a few minutes to complete your next self-evaluation on the subject of fat management in order to pinpoint some areas you can focus on. The last two pages of this chapter include two charts that will help you estimate the number of calories you burn in various activities.

Hopefully you took the initial evaluations in chapter 2. Now, after reading this chapter, you may see these same questions with a little more insight. Your answers will most likely be the same for now. Change will occur as you apply these principles. Take this evaluation again and every couple months to gauge your journey toward victory!

— Lifestyle Evaluation—Fat Management

Based on the past three months, please rate yourself (0–Almost never; 1–Sometimes; 2–Often; 3–Always).

_____ I feel in control of my food choices.

_____ I measure my size by how I look and feel, not the scale.

_____ I eat only when I'm hungry.

_____ I stop eating when I'm full.

_____ I understand why calories count.

_____ I eat four to five small meals or snacks per day.

_____ I limit my junk food, fast food, and desserts to less than 15 percent of my diet.

_____ I am happy with my body weight.

_____ I am happy with my size and shape.

_____ I can enjoy "fun food" without feeling guilty.

_____ I think about food only when I'm hungry.

_____ I can see myself eating and living in control.

_____ I walk or get purposeful exercise at least four times per week.

_____ I am very aware of my choices and how they affect my body.

_____ I say no to the latest diets or supplements promising quick results.

_____ I know if I'm going to be lean, I have to take daily action.

_____ Add the total of all scores.

Scoring

40–48 Excellent! You've got a lean lifestyle.

31–39 Good. You're doing most things right!

22–30 Fair. It's time to take action.

< 21 Poor. Start with one step at a time.

— Fat Management Menu

——— *Increase Your Daily Calorie Burn*

Aerobic activity is number one

An active lifestyle makes a difference

Wear Caltrac—your personal activity coach

——— *Decrease Your Daily Calorie Intake*

Read labels

Find enjoyable substitutions

Count calories for absolute truth

Keep a food diary

Use portion control
Plan your snacks
Shop for success
Cut your losses

Get a Handle on Emotional Eating

Identify your triggers
Create new habits
Tune into the hunger scale
Legalize foods
Bury diet attitudes
Learn to cut your losses

Increase Your Energy and Metabolism

Practice the NutriMax Six (see Nutrition Menu in chapter 12)
Never eat less than your RMR
Fuel and burn all day long

Practice Healthy Thinking

Identify your lies
Rewrite your self-talk
Listen to your tapes
Practice trigger talk

My Fat Management Recipe

Priority	Action
#1 _____	_____
	_____
	_____

#2 _____   _____

                             _____

                             _____

#3 _____   _____

                             _____

                             _____

#4 _____   _____

                             _____

                             _____

Hints on Conceptualizing Calories

Understand what a "serving" is (refer to page 221).

When in doubt, measure.

Read labels and interpret them accurately.

Equate serving sizes with everyday items, such as:

A deck of cards = three oz. of meat, poultry, or fish

Your fist = one cup of rice, potatoes, pasta, or medium fruit

Your thumb = one oz. of cheese or candy

Calorie Burn Chart

Based on a 130-pound woman

ACTIVITY (based on a 130-pound woman)	15 minutes	30	45	60
Aerobics (high-impact)	104	207	311	414
Aerobics (low-impact)	74	148	222	296
Ballet	89	177	266	354
Bicycling (12 to 14 mph)	118	236	354	472
Box aerobics	133	265	398	530
Circuit weight training	118	236	354	472
Cross-country skiing	150	300	450	600
Downhill skiing	74	148	222	296

201

Golf (carrying clubs)	81	162	243	324
In-line skating	104	207	311	414
Jumping rope (moderate)	148	295	443	590
Kayaking	74	148	222	296
Mountain biking	126	251	377	502
Racquetball	104	207	311	414
Rowing machine	150	300	450	600
Running (8.5-minute mile)	170	339	509	678
Ski machine	140	280	320	560
Slide (moderate)	101	201	302	402
Stair climber	105	210	315	420
Stationary biking (vigorous)	155	310	465	620
Step aerobics	169	337	506	674
Swimming				
(crawl, 50 yards per minute)	143	285	428	570
Tennis (singles)	118	236	354	472
VersaClimber	161	322	483	644
Walking (12-minute mile)	113	225	413	550
(15-minute mile, flat)	88	175	263	350
(20-minute mile, flat)	63	125	188	250
(20-minute mile, 4 percent incline)	100	200	300	400
Water aerobics	59	118	177	236
Weight lifting (vigorous)	89	177	266	354
Yoga	59	118	177	236

Calorie Burn Chart
Based on a 180-pound man

ACTIVITY (based on a 180-pound man)	15 minutes	30	45	60
Aerobics (high-impact)	135	269	404	538
Aerobics (low-impact)	96	192	289	385
Ballet	116	230	346	460
Bicycling (12 to 14 mph)	153	307	460	614
Box aerobics	173	345	517	689
Circuit weight training	153	307	460	614
Cross-country skiing	195	390	585	780
Downhill skiing	96	192	289	385
Golf (carrying clubs)	105	211	316	421
In-line skating	135	269	404	538
Jumping rope (moderate)	192	384	576	767
Kayaking	96	192	289	385
Mountain biking	164	326	490	653
Racquetball	135	269	404	538
Rowing machine	195	390	585	780
Running (8.5-minute mile)	221	441	662	881

Ski machine	182	364	416	728
Slide (moderate)	131	261	393	523
Stair climber	136	273	410	546
Stationary biking (vigorous)	202	403	605	806
Step aerobics	220	438	658	876
Swimming				
(crawl, 50 yards per minute)	186	371	556	741
Tennis (singles)	153	307	460	614
VersaClimber	209	419	628	837
Walking (12-minute mile)	147	293	537	715
(15-minute mile, flat)	114	228	344	458
(20-minute mile, flat)	82	163	244	325
(20-minute mile, 4 percent incline)	130	260	390	520
Water aerobics	77	153	230	307
Weight lifting (vigorous)	116	230	346	460
Yoga	77	153	230	307

— 12
—— you are
— what you eat

I read a story about an elderly carpenter who told his employer that he was getting ready to retire. His boss, the contractor, was sad to lose him and asked if he could build just one more house as a personal favor. The carpenter said yes. Unfortunately, it was obvious his heart was not in his work as he cut corners and built with little attention to detail. When the house was done, the employer handed the key to the carpenter as his retirement gift. The old man had no idea he was building the house for himself, and now he had to live in the home he had carelessly thrown together.

We are the "carpenters" of our bodies. Over time, all the cells in our bodies will be replaced with new ones. Skin and blood cells change quickly; others, such as our bones, take longer. In total, we have a completely new body, including our skeleton, every seven years. We are in essence building our new "homes" one meal at a time. Build wisely. Your body tomorrow will be the result of the choices you make today.

— Imagine Your Body as a Car

Like cars, our bodies need regular, quality fuel to run effectively. Since most of us like food, we want our cars to burn a lot of fuel. So in this example, imagine your car is a Ferrari—a sleek, fast-burning, high-performance Ferrari.

What kind of fuel would you put in that kind of car? Premium, high-octane fuel is the best, of course! Now if your car held sixteen gallons, and you put in fifteen gallons of premium fuel and only one gallon of regular, how would it run? It would probably run fairly well, since the largest percentage of fuel is premium. But what if you put in half premium fuel and half regular? I'm sure the performance would be compromised. That's how it is with your body as well. It can take a little regular (or empty calories) now and then, as long it is getting quality fuel most of the time. Unfortunately, many Americans eat more "fun food" than nutritious food, and then they wonder why they feel like they have chronic fatigue syndrome.

Most of you don't need an advanced course in nutrition. Micromanaging your nutrition is like getting your car tuned up with new filters and spark plugs but never filling up the gas tank with quality fuel. What we need is to be reminded of the basics and understand how certain foods can "rev" up our engine for high energy. It is far better to improve your nutrition 10 or 20 percent for a lifetime than to eat "perfectly" for a few short months and revert back to your old habits.

— Simple Truths

—— *My Basic Philosophy*

Nutrition is a "soft" science. We have a lot of information about food and how our bodies work, but there are also a lot of different opinions about how best to use the information. For the sake of simplicity, let me explain my basic philosophy.

If it were so difficult to eat and live healthfully, I really believe God would have given us an extensive user's manual. Think about it. How did we survive for thousands of years without all this nutritional research, special studies, and books? In simpler times, people ate the foods available to them. Fat-free cookies, cakes, and other treats didn't grow on trees. It's unlikely that cavemen found anything closely resembling a white bagel or pasta in the average cave, either.

While the human body has changed very little over thousands of years, our dietary habits have changed dramatically . . . and not for the better! Hundreds of years ago, people had no choice but to eat food the way God created it. Chocolate chip cookies and corn chips weren't on his list, and the greatest extravagance probably was the occasional feast on a fatted calf. And in days past, the average person burned thousands of calories each day just surviving. Today our fingers, using all of our high-tech conveniences, get more exercise than our feet.

Now, I am not a nutritional perfectionist, although I could teach *you* how to be one. I just don't believe it is necessary to throw every single empty calorie out of your diet. I have my own weaknesses. I simply love my Starbucks decaf latte with one "pump" of mocha, which I enjoy several times a week. And a small taste of something sweet after a meal is another indulgence I satisfy on occasion as well. The key to good health and effective fat management is the frequency and amount of the compromises you allow in your daily diet.

I believe it is possible to nourish your body for excellent health and still enjoy food for pure pleasure, if done in moderation. It is a matter of balance. Try to eat as much natural food as you can as frequently as possible. If you could actually see what is happening inside your body when you eat too much sugar, white flour, and saturated fat, you would be shocked! We need to retrain our minds and taste buds to crave and enjoy natural foods more than all the decadent snacks we have come to love.

—— *Eating for High Energy, Low Body Fat, and Maximum Health*

It's pretty simple to eat right. Most of us just need to get back to the basics. You know, all the stuff your mom used to tell you, like, "Eat your fruits and veggies. Drink lots of water. Go easy on the junk food." I love what Dr. James Balch says in his book *The Super Antioxidants:*

> When God created humans, He also provided all the nutrients we needed to maintain a healthy body. He did not hide those nutrients from us, and He didn't package them separately and write a book to explain exactly how each one functions. He simply put an abundance of nutrients in the foods that we would eat.[1]

I couldn't agree more. Just take some time to ponder all the variety of foods God has created. In fact, tear open a juicy orange, bite into a delicious nectarine, or peel a ripe banana and marvel at how anyone could doubt there is a divine Creator! Man has never come close to packaging food as perfectly as our God has. And to top it off, we are still discovering in plant foods a multitude of micronutrients called phytochemicals that we didn't even know existed. These powerhouse nutrients prevent cancer, balance hormones, and slow down aging. No man-made foods or supplements will ever match the perfect balance found in God's own recipe for nutrition.

There are two basic nutritional components: macronutrients and micronutrients. Macronutrients provide calories in the form of carbohydrates, protein, and fat, and are the only nutrients the body can metabolize for energy. Micronutrients are noncaloric and include vitamins, minerals, and phytochemicals. Micronutrients cannot give you extra energy, but they do help with the process of metabolizing energy.

The following recommendations are considered reasonable ranges for most people. The ideal blend for you may vary from day to day. Through trial and error, you will learn to eat according to your body's individual responses. I have given you ranges referenced as both percentages of total caloric intake as well as an example of total grams based on a two-thousand-calorie model below:

Ideal Ranges of Macronutrients

Carbohydrates: 45–60 percent Carbohydrates: 225–300 g
Proteins: 15–30 percent Proteins: 75–150 g
Fats: 15–25 percent Fats: 33–55 g

Carbohydrates and fats are the body's preferred sources of fuel for energy. Protein's more important function is the building and repairing of body tissues. It is converted to energy only when carbohydrates and fats aren't available. That's why people on restrictive, low-calorie diets lose muscle mass. The mix of carbohydrate, proteins, and fat in our diets has a powerful impact on how we feel and how long we are satisfied after eating. Try to include each of these three elements in every meal or snack, with a higher concentration of protein early in the day.

To improve your energy, health, and fat management, you need to address the essentials. I call them the NutriMax Six. But before we delve into those, a word of wisdom before you get too excited. Don't overwhelm yourself by taking on too much. At the end of the chapter, you will have an opportunity to evaluate your nutritional habits and design a plan to *begin* some new lifestyle habits. Determine what two or three things are the most important or what you can handle right now. Start there and add more changes as you are ready.

— The NutriMax Six

—— #1—Water

Second only to air, your body must have a constant supply of water to survive. Most people die of dehydration within a few days without it. Your body doesn't sweat soda or iced tea; it sweats water and electrolytes. It needs water to perform all of its bodily functions, and when you don't drink enough, it resorts to handling only the most essential functions first . . . and that is not metabolizing excess fat! Try to drink at least four to eight ounces of water for every hour you are awake. If you wait to drink it until you're thirsty, you're already a quart low (four cups). If you want to look younger, have more energy, and live longer, drink pure, fresh water all day long!

—— #2—Plant Foods

Fiber-rich fruits, vegetables, whole grains, beans, legumes, seeds, and nuts are packed with phytochemicals, antioxidants, and fiber. All three help fight cancer, provide anti-aging protection, and more. Mom was right to encourage you to eat more of these foods. Now that you're not under her watchful eye, how are you doing on your own? And if you are a mom, how are your kids doing? The old recommendation to have seven to nine fruit and vegetable servings today is still great advice. When was the last time you even came close? It's tough, even on a good day.

Study after study shows increasing evidence that this area of nutrition will have the most profound long-term effect on your health and vitality. Supplements cannot completely fill in the gaps left from not eating enough whole foods. The fiber alone in plant foods has an incredible balancing effect on blood sugar, not to mention the benefits to your entire digestive system. And don't forget that your breads and cereals should have enough whole grains to be considered food. Most refined, packaged foods enter the body and are pretty much turned to sugar and paste within minutes of ingestion. Wonder why you feel so sluggish?

#3—Protein

Protein is essential for tissue repair, maintenance, and growth of muscles, blood, hormones, enzymes, and antibodies. You should always eat some protein with breakfast and lunch, because protein digests very slowly, stabilizes your blood sugar, and makes you feel satiated longer. However, more is not always better. Too much protein can overtax your body, particularly wreaking havoc on your kidneys. There is absolutely no healthful evidence to validate the outrageous propensity toward high-protein diets. Why did God create such an incredible array of colorful foods for us to eat if we were designed to be predominately carnivores? More about *that* later! For now, try to get at least twelve to fourteen grams of protein at both breakfast and lunch. Also, find creative ways to add a little protein to your snacks, such as nuts, peanut butter on whole grain crackers, and so on. (That's right . . . nuts! Yes, I know they are high in fat—good fat. Eat them in moderation, and you can enjoy both the taste and the health benefits.)

#4—Fats

Choosing the right fats and understanding their benefits and drawbacks will help you dramatically in your weight management efforts. Keeping the right amount of healthy fat in your diet will leave you feeling full and satiated longer than a nonfat meal. Fats have long been getting a bad rap, but the truth is that some are essential to your health. The key is to eat the right kind because, as with carbohydrates, not all are created equal. Lots of people simply eat too much fat. But many more get almost none of the vitally essential omega-3 fatty acids that have a crucial impact on our health. This essential fat dramatically impacts

211

brain function and cardiac health and has been linked to positive protection from Alzheimer's disease. For now, try to reduce the saturated (animal and dairy) fats as much as possible. The total fat in your diet should range between 15 and 30 percent, so stay on the lower end until you reach your ideal size. Olive oil is always a good choice for cooking and salads. Or try adding omega-3 fats to your diet by eating cold-water fish like salmon and tuna at least two times per week. Walnuts and flaxseed are also very high in omega-3 fat.

───── #5—Vitamins, Minerals, and Antioxidants

Vitamins and minerals are nutrients that occur naturally in foods and are essential for health yet provide no calories. Antioxidants are a specific group of nutrients that form an army to capture the metabolic waste products called free radicals and transport them out of the body before they can damage the cells. All these micronutrients act like spark plugs, working to help the body do its various functions effectively. They also help us more effectively utilize our food as fuel and prevent nutritional deficiencies.

God provides all the nutrients we need in natural foods. The problem is that we don't eat the amount and variety of whole foods necessary to meet all of our nutritional needs. We also have corrupted our natural food sources with depleted soil, polluted water, and chemical agents like pesticides.

Today, it's important to take vitamins and minerals as an insurance policy. However, they do not take the place of healthy eating. New spark plugs won't make your car run better if you forget to put gasoline in your car. And vitamins without good food are of little value.

If you're not already taking vitamins, start with a good multivitamin mineral complex and an antioxidant formula. Then, if you have a specific need, supplement based on the recommendations of your health-care professional. A word of wisdom: Don't spend a fortune on micromanaging your nutrition before you get the basics down. Make the NutriMax Six a consistent habit, then start fine-tuning.

—— #6—*Vitamins Z and X*

Vitamin Z—better known as sleep—is another frequently neglected "nutrient" that plays a much more important role in our health than people have previously realized. And Vitamin X—better known as exercise—is essential for maintaining high energy, low body fat, and overall health and vitality. Okay, okay . . . I know neither are technically nutrients. But if these two lifestyle factors are not a high priority, even perfect nutrition will not bring you the health, vitality, and fast-burning metabolism you desire.

Sleep is the time when you get both physical and psychological rest. During deep sleep, your body accomplishes its most important cellular renewal. Even modest amounts of sleep deprivation can diminish your immune system and ability to cope with the daily challenges of life. If you want to look younger, feel better, and live longer—get enough sleep! How much is enough? Experts suggest that most people need close to eight hours of sleep every night.

I have found that chronic fatigue is one of the biggest factors impacting an out-of-control appetite. I think the body is saying, "If you're not going to give me enough quality rest to reenergize, I'm just going to beg for sugar and calories all day long to make up for it!" My suggestion: Make sleep a priority. Try getting eight hours of sleep a night for a full month and see the impact it makes in your lifestyle.

Exercise will be covered fully in chapter 14. For now, let me leave you with an important thought that will motivate you to move more. Exercise is an incredible energizer. The more you move, the better you feel. Feeling good motivates you to stay active, and activity tends to distract you from sedentary habits that include eating. Get in a positive cycle and get a good dose of Vitamin X every day!

— The NutriZap Four

While legalizing foods is a healthy emotional approach to take, we must admit that too many empty calories are bad for our health. I define these empty-calorie foods as "pure pleasure/no value." But the good news is that there is a balance between legalizing and limiting fun foods.

Because I host a weekly health show, I have the privilege of interviewing many dynamic health professionals. One of my favorites is Dr. Francisco Contreras. In his book *A Healthy Heart*, he states that the top three staples of the American diet are (1) refined sugar, (2) refined flour, and (3) processed oils.

He states, "Many of our foods have become so processed, preserved and chemicalized that they are hardly foods at all, but rather manufactured products that happen to be somewhat digestible."[2]

Designing your nutritional lifestyle does not require perfection. But it is very important to plan strategically for moderate indulgences in your diet without compromising your health or waistline. It goes back to the car analogy. If 10 to 15 percent of your "fuel" is low-grade processed foods such as cookies, chips, even white bread, your car will still perform pretty well. For example, a large, 250-calorie chocolate chip cookie would do it for one day. But as the percentage of junk goes up, your energy and wellness go down, down, down!

While following the six NutriMax principles will definitely charge up your body for high-energy fat burning, there are four mainstays of the American diet that will run your engine down. I call them the NutriZap Four. Let's take a quick look at the "zappers."

— #1—Sugar

Sugar tastes good to your taste buds and acts badly in your body. Simply stated: Sugar is not good for you. Whether it's sucrose, fructose, lactose, raw, confectioners, or "natural" . . . to your body, it all translates to sugar. I explained earlier that your brain needs a constant supply of glucose to survive, but that doesn't mean you need to ingest sugar in its simplest form. Our bodies are great at converting any kind of food to sugar in order to provide an ample supply of glucose to our brains. In fact, refined sugar has only been part of our diets since the mid-1700s.

According to Dr. James Balch in his latest book, *The Super Antioxidants,* when excess sugar reacts with proteins in the body, it produces a damaging effect similar to the free radicals we've heard so much about in recent years. Sugar promotes aging, decreases your immunity, promotes weight gain, and increases your incidence of diseases like diabetes.[3]

Of course, this doesn't mean that you have to throw all sweet foods out of your life forever. But it is highly recommended that you treat yourself very modestly with high-sugar foods and beverages. I follow a couple of personal rules that I think work very well. I almost never have anything sweet before lunch. I don't drink any beverages with sugar or fructose. And I keep my desserts or other sweet selections to no more than about two hundred to three hundred calories per day.

Now that doesn't mean I have dessert every day! By holding off on eating your sugary foods until late in the day, you protect yourself from big blood sugar swings that destroy your energy. And when your energy is high, you tend to have fewer cravings for sweets anyway.

—— #2—*White Flour*

White bagels, white rice, and white-flour pastas convert very quickly to sugar. In fact, if you put a piece of white bread in your mouth for a few minutes, you will notice a sweet taste. The starch is converting to glucose. Yes, your white bread is fortified with important vitamins and minerals, such as iron and folic acid, and contains a smidgen of protein and fiber. But for the most part, refined carbohydrates are sweet nothings. Think of it this way: Every slice of white bread you eat is a bit like eating three or four vitamin-fortified marshmallows. A cup of pasta? Eight marshmallows. A "marshmallow" diet can make a big difference in your health.

Have you ever mixed a little water into a big bowl of white flour? What do you get? Paste! And that is what too many crackers and other processed foods are becoming in your digestive tract. It may sound extreme, but I label French bread, white bagels, and saltines right up there with other junk food like chips, cookies, and cakes!

Back in 1978, John Weisburger, M.D., Ph.D., noted that the American people would be better off if the FDA banned white bread! Hmmm. I think this is too important to ignore. My advice is to start replacing half or more of your refined carbohydrates with healthier, disease-preventing whole grain carbohydrates.

—— #3—"Bad" Fat

If you were to get your blood drawn right after a fatty meal, you would be horrified. You can actually see the fat in the tube of blood as it comes out of your vein! Sometimes I wish that God had given us little personal scopes to see what was happening microscopically in our bodies in response to our lifestyle habits. I truly believe it would motivate us to stop doing some things and start doing others.

The point is that most of us are eating way too much saturated and "trans" fat. All those years we were eating margarine and thinking we were doing the "right thing," and we were actually deceiving ourselves! As it turns out, when vegetable oil is hydrogenated to be solid at room temperature, it produces "trans fats" that act much like saturated fats. The problem is that we are getting unhealthy fat from a multitude of sources. The obvious source is meat and dairy products. But much of the fat is

216

hidden in our packaged foods. Become an unhealthy fat detective and start getting some of that sludge out of your diet today!

—— *#4—Caffeine*

Is caffeine the perfect early morning "pick me upper"? Yes and no. Caffeine is a central nervous system stimulant. The reason it jump-starts you in the morning or reenergizes you in the afternoon is because it stimulates your body to produce adrenaline, the stress hormone. It raises your pulse, increases your breathing, and sometimes even raises your blood pressure. Two hundred milligrams of caffeine is enough to make some people feel nervous and raise their blood pressure two to three points. And I don't know anyone who needs any more stress hormone stimulation.

Most experts agree that two cups of coffee per day (or the equivalent amount of caffeine in other beverages) is fairly safe for most people. It can slightly increase your mental clarity and definitely improve wakefulness. Of course, the flip side is that caffeine can delay the onset of sleep and interfere with rapid eye movement (REM) sleep, the stage when people dream. Caffeine reaches peak concentration in the bloodstream within thirty to sixty minutes, and it takes approximately four to six hours for its effects to wear off.

In the big picture, caffeine ultimately "deenergizes" you. Once the adrenaline effect wears off, your energy, hydration levels, and even blood sugar begin to dip. The natural reaction is to crave more coffee or sugar again. And if you take on too much caffeine, you end up totally zapped of energy by the end of the day. So if you really want to be a high-energy person, forego the caffeine, at least until after lunch, and drink lots of water.

Another great reason to remove caffeine from your diet is because it robs you of calcium. So my latte rich in calcium would be wiped out nutritionally if I indulged in caffeinated coffee. An easy rule of thumb is to drink a cup of milk or eat two tablespoons of yogurt for each cup of caffeinated coffee you drink. If you love the taste of coffee, the operative word is *decaf.*

— Nutritional Poisons

In addition, you may want to consider reducing or eliminating some harmful elements from your diet, which include chemicals, preservatives, and "synthetic" foods. Our bodies were not designed to ingest foreign substances. It is impossible to know the long-term effect that things like artificial sweeteners and fat-alternative products will have on our health. But for example, in recent decades the incidence of cancer in children and young adults has been staggering. You have to wonder how much nutrition is impacting our futures!

—— *Fake Fats*

Olestra (Olean) is a synthetic fat that's used to fry chips without the usual artery clogging, waist-expanding fat. Does that sound too good to be true? Experts say it is. According to Meir J. Stampfer, M.D., a Harvard researcher, the problem with olestra is twofold. First, since olestra passes through the body undigested, it can cause severe and incapacitating diarrhea, loose stools, abdominal cramps, and flatulence. Second, it can deplete the body of crucial fat-soluble vitamins (A, D, E, and K). It also reduces the body's absorption of fat-soluble carotenoids (antioxidant compounds such as alpha- and beta-carotene, lycopene, and lutein) from fruits and vegetables.

Stampfer estimates that over the next decade, olestra consumption could cause up to 9,800 additional cases of prostate cancer, 32,000 additional cases of coronary artery disease, and 7,400 additional cases of lung cancer *each year.* Companies producing olestra products maintain it is safe, and the FDA seems to agree. However, my opinion is to just enjoy a little real fat on occasion, forget the fake stuff, and move on.

—— *Artificial Sweeteners*

The most widely known artificial sweeteners are aspartame and saccharin. You'll find these in "diet" foods like frozen desserts, soft drinks, chewing gum, gelatin, no-sugar-added baked goods, and tabletop sweeteners.

Many studies are showing that these products actually increase our sugar cravings. Most nutritionists, including our Patti Milligan, R.D., M.S., recommend taking in a few extra calories and ingesting the real thing. A study done at Harvard and other medical centers in the Boston area in the 1980s found that eating saccharin was the single most reliable predictor of weight gain.

Saccharin (Sweet'n Low) is 350 times sweeter than sugar. Studies show that it can cause cancer of the bladder, uterus, ovaries, skin, blood vessels, and other organs. It also appears to increase the potency of other cancer-causing chemicals. Yuck!

Aspartame (Equal) has generated more FDA complaints than any other additive on the market. There are actually three rooms full of boxes for this sweetener alone! Aspartame does cross the "blood-brain" barrier, which means it can get directly into circulation in our brains. People who use aspartame have reported a variety of symptoms including dizziness, hallucinations, headaches, forgetfulness, fatigue, and the like. Sounds like we should probably avoid it completely.

But there is a healthful, noncaloric alternative—Stevia. This is a natural sweetener made from chrysanthemums that has almost no calories and no known side effects or dangers. At present, it can be purchased in health food stores as a sweetener, but it is not currently released to be used as an additive in foods. Patti Milligan does recommend this sugar substitute.

—— *Additives, Pesticides, and All the Other "Junk"*

Eating nutritiously in this day and age can be a challenge. Many professionals agree that the pesticides, hormones, and additives in our diets are the culprits behind many diseases and health challenges, and these things can be especially harmful to children. Whenever possible, shop for hormone-free meats and poultry. Invest a little extra in organic fruits and vegetables. Pay more attention to food labels. By increasing the quality of your overall diet with nutritious whole foods and lots of pure, fresh water, you are supporting your body's ability to neutralize and remove these toxins quickly.

You don't have to become a fanatic to maintain a healthy body. But it does help to tune in to the potential junk you are ingesting on a regular or periodic basis. Become aware and start making little shifts in your nutritional habits. Your body will thank you!

— Learn to Read Labels

Now that you have a better handle on what to eat, you need to be able to discern what's inside those packages you're pulling off the grocery store shelves. You'll be amazed at what you can learn (and how your choices will change) when you take the time to read the labels on all your potential purchases. Don't assume all similar foods have the same components. Reading labels accurately is essential, because it is important to make choices based on complete information. Check out the sample label on the next page and look for these things:

Serving Size. Always check the serving size first. If you eat more or less, you must adjust your calories accordingly.

Daily Value. This tells you how much of a day's worth of fat, sodium, calories, etc., the food provides based on a two-thousand-calorie diet. It does not tell you the actual percentage in the food item. (You must calculate that for yourself.)

```
                    Nutrition Facts
      Serving Size 12 oz. (340g)
      Servings Per Container 1
                  Amount Per Serving
      Calories 340          Calories from Fat 45
                              % Daily Value*
      Total Fat 5g                      8%
       Saturated Fat 2g                10%
        Cholesterol 30mg               10%
      Sodium 470mg                     20%
      Total Carbohydrate 61g           20%
       Dietary Fiber 5g                20%
       Sugars 2-3g
      Protein 14g
      Vitamin A 10%        Vitamin C  35%
      Calcium  15%         Iron       10%

      *Percent Daily Values are based on a 2,000-calorie
      diet. Your daily values may be higher or lower
      depending on your calorie needs:
                          Calories:        2,000
      Total Fat            65g             80g
      Sat Fat              20g             25g
      Cholesterol          300mg           300mg
      Sodium               2,400mg         2,400mg
      Total Carbohydrate   300g            375g
      Dietary Fiber        25g             30g
      Calories per gram:
      Fat 9 • Carbohydrate 4 • Protein 4
```

Calories from Fat. Now you can see just how many calories are coming from fat. You will have to do the math to compute the actual percentages. An easy rule of thumb is:

15 percent fat = 1.5 grams per 100 calories

20 percent fat = 2.0 grams per 100 calories

25 percent fat = 2.5 grams per 100 calories

Carbohydrates and Sugar. Become aware of the composition of your food. High-sugar foods will promote blood sugar instability.

Fiber. Choose foods with a higher fiber content, which will slow down carbohydrate absorption. In processed foods and packaged cereals, choose foods with a minimum of two to four grams of fiber per serving. There are a few cereals with six to eight grams per serving . . . even better!

Protein. Become aware of your protein sources. Did you get 15 to 30 percent protein in your diet today?

221

Read every product label before you purchase the food. And if there are labels on most of your foods, you aren't eating enough whole, natural stuff. Shop first where you find foods closer to how God originally created them. Always make eating nutritiously your first priority. Try to eat a healthful mix of foods, with a special emphasis on lots of fruits and vegetables, and balance your carbohydrates, proteins, and fats to meet your body's specific needs. You can tell when you have found the right blend—your body will respond with high energy.

Remember, you build a completely new body every seven years, and it can only be as strong as the supplies you give it to work with. You really are what you eat! As you make decisions about how you will eat and live for a lifetime, remember that you can't build a brick house out of straw, nor can you build a healthy body out of sugar.

— Fuel and Burn All Day Long

Eating for health and energy should start to become more important than simply getting the fat off our bodies. But we do want to make sure that goal is accomplished as well. With this in mind, remember what I taught you in chapter 11 about eating and burning all day long as if you were a car with a five-gallon tank.

Your body actually knows about how many calories it needs at specific times of day. If you don't fuel up right, it revolts with fatigue, cravings, and more efficient fat storage. But if you eat and burn all day long with more frequent yet smaller meals and snacks, your body will respond with higher energy because it has sufficient, immediate fuel throughout the day.

When we start seeing pounds sneak on our bodies, our first instinct is often to skip meals. Don't! As you learned earlier, cutting calories too dramatically can damage your metabolism. Even if you eat the same number of calories, you'll burn them off better if you spread them throughout the day.

This is especially true for postmenopausal women, who find it easier to put weight on and harder to take it off. Research from Tufts University in Boston suggests that after age fifty, women who eat larger meals instead of nutritious mini-meals may burn off sixty fewer calories a day. That means switching to mini-meals, spaced throughout the day, could save you from gaining six pounds a year.

—— *Begin with Breakfast*

Breakfast is the most important meal of the day. It stimulates your metabolism to get cooking early in the day and sets the stage for your energy level in the afternoon. In fact, studies show breakfast increases your metabolism by about 10 percent. That's huge!

What is a good breakfast? Always include a strong base of complex carbohydrates (full of fiber) that act as kindling to stoke your metabolic fire, balanced with moderate amounts of protein and smaller amounts of fat. Periodically stoking your fire all day long with this blend of foods will enhance your calorie-burning capability.

Overeating diverts large amounts of blood to your digestive tract and makes you feel sleepy and sluggish. That is why you get the "after-lunch blahs." So get lean and energized by eating more of your calories in the first twelve hours of your day when you burn them best! Try to avoid refined carbohydrates, sugars, and caffeine until after lunch when you have created a strong nutritional base of protein and fiber to stabilize your blood sugar. Begin to practice this discipline consistently, and it will help sugar cravings become a thing of the past.

—— *Seven Small Steps You Can Take Right Now*

1. Don't try to micromanage your nutrition. Get the basics down first.

223

2. Eat as well as you can every day by practicing the Nutri-Max Six.
3. Keep supplementation simple. More is not always better.
4. Listen to your body—it will tell you how you are doing.
5. Seek professional help if you aren't at peak health.
6. Keep a reasonable and healthy perspective.
7. Remember, every small improvement counts!

— But Wait, There's More!

For those of you who are intrigued about learning more specifics about nutrition, the remaining information in this chapter is for you. But even if you choose to stop reading here and simply begin adding the NutriMax Six into your lifestyle and decreasing the NutriZappers, you will notice significant improvements in your energy and long-term health. Just don't skip the self-evaluation of your current nutritional habits at the end of this chapter.

—— *Wonderful Water*

Water is life! It is the number one nutritional factor. After all, we can only survive for about forty-eight hours without it. I have interviewed scores of people, and low water intake is the most common reason for low energy. Just imagine that each cell in your body is like a grape. When you don't drink enough water, your cells begin to look like raisins. Do you want your skin or muscle cells to look like raisins?

Your muscle tissue is about 75 percent water, and your blood is about 90 percent water. When you don't drink enough, your body becomes less efficient at transporting nutrients to all the cells in your body and carrying waste products from the cells to the kidneys for excretion in urine. Your body also needs water to:

- digest your food
- lubricate your joints
- create a protective cushion around your organs and tissues, including the eyes and spinal cord
- metabolize fat
- regulate your body's temperature through sweating

Your body will always deal with the most important bodily functions first. It needs sufficient water to do its work, so you should drink at least eight to ten glasses a day and more on days you exercise, due to increased sweating and breathing. Here's why: The average person loses ten cups of water per day—two cups to sweating and evaporation, two cups to breathing, and six cups to waste removal. You can replace up to two cups through the water in the foods you eat, but you have to make up the remaining eight cups by drinking fluids, preferably pure water.

Dehydration causes numerous symptoms including fatigue, poor concentration, headaches, blurred vision, and lack of neuromuscular control. When you are hungry, start off with a glass of fresh water. If you're feeling low on energy or if something hurts (like a headache), drink a glass of water. If you wait to drink water until you are thirsty, you are already dehydrated. So drink at least four to eight ounces every hour you're awake, whether you feel like it or not.

The best way to develop a water habit is to have it with you at all times—in your car, at your desk, at the bathroom sink when you're getting ready in the morning. Carry your water bottle with you everywhere and drink up!

—— *Plant Foods*

Potatoes, tomatoes, onions, and iceberg lettuce. The four most popular vegetables in the United States often end up as french fries, potato chips, on pizza and in ketchup, or on Big Macs and Whoppers. Make no mistake. There's no such thing as a bad vegetable. All fruits and vegetables have nutritional benefits. Most are loaded with fiber, vitamins, and some minerals. But how do we choose the best from all the good? The key health-promoting nutrients that researchers encourage us to eat more of are carotenoids (beta-carotene and others), folic acid (the B vitamins), potassium, vitamin C, calcium, and fiber.

Fruits are generally quite low in calcium, but the top ten fruits that supply the highest quantity of carotenoids, folic acid, potassium, vitamin C, and fiber are (in order):

1. Guava
2. Watermelon
3. Grapefruit (pink or red)
4. Kiwi
5. Papaya
6. Cantaloupe
7. Apricots (dried)
8. Oranges
9. Strawberries
10. Blackberries

These vegetables supply the highest quantity of carotenoids, folic acid, potassium, vitamin C, and fiber, plus calcium:

1. Collard greens
2. Spinach
3. Kale
4. Swiss chard
5. Red pepper
6. Sweet potatoes
7. Pumpkin (canned)
8. Carrots

9. Broccoli

10. Okra

Fresh produce tastes wonderful when in season, so experiment with all the color, crunch, and leafy greens. Don't forget to check the frozen section in the grocery store when fresh produce is not available. Frozen fruits and vegetables are preserved at the peak of their nutritional value, and some contain just as many nutrients as fresh produce—sometimes more, depending on how long the fresh ones have sat on display or in a refrigerator. And canned is better than nothing. (Note: Many products have added sugar, so buy unsweetened frozen and canned fruits. Also, rinse canned vegetables to reduce the sodium content.)

As I say week after week on my radio show, *Healthy Solutions*, there is an endless supply of information about why we should get passionate about eating seven to nine fruits and vegetables each and every day for the rest of our lives! And when we can't (or don't), there are some great supplements that can help us fill in the gaps.

But man will never be able to replicate what God has done perfectly, which is to package food in exact formulations to nourish us completely. Plant foods provide you with protecting phytochemicals, which can dramatically impact your overall health. For example, garlic contains a substance called alliin, a natural antibiotic. Indoles can be found in cabbage and broccoli. These help protect against cancer. Dried beans and peas are full of saponins, which help lower cholesterol and protect against osteoporosis. Tomatoes contain the richest source of the phytochemical lycopene, the pigment that gives them their red color. You'll notice that one glass of tomato juice has the lycopene of forty tomato slices! Take a look at the top ten list again and shoot for the most nutrient-packed, phytochemical vegetables you can find.

Every second of your life, your cells are bombarded by dangerous particles called free radicals. Free radicals are molecules that are missing an electron, which they attempt to snatch from any other molecule available. In a split second, they can alter your DNA in ways that cause cancer, change LDL cholesterol (the bad cholesterol) so it sticks to artery walls, or damage collagen and make skin wrinkle prone. The oxidation effect can be compared to the browning of a cut apple or the rust on a car. You cannot see or feel the damage of these free radicals until many cells are compromised and disease or premature aging results.

Fortunately, you can fight back. Load your diet with antioxidants—the natural zappers of free radicals—by eating lots of fruits and vegetables. The bright and dark color of fruits and vegetables generally means they are richer in nutrients. For example, buy red grapes instead of green, red cabbage instead of green, and romaine lettuce instead of iceberg.

Here's an interesting fact about antioxidants. Tufts University in Boston and scientist Ronald Prior, Ph.D., recommend adding a half cup of blueberries to your diet every day (a dramatic increase over our current average intake of about two and a half cups a year). With a half cup of blueberries, you can practically double the amount of antioxidants most Americans get in one day. Blueberries beat out thirty-nine other common fruits and vegetables in antioxidant power—even kale, strawberries, spinach, and broccoli! Wow!

Buy produce at different stages of ripeness so there will always be some ready for you to eat. Splurge on prepackaged salads, fruits, and vegetables. They might be a little more expensive, but they're time efficient and you're more likely to eat the produce before it goes bad in your refrigerator. Just think of it as an investment in your health. Make it a practice to buy one new kind of healthful food every time you go to the supermarket.

—— *Fiber*

In centuries past, the base of people's diets looked much different than today. It contained large amounts of fiber, one of the most neglected elements of the American diet. The average person only eats about ten to fifteen grams of fiber per day. We need an absolute minimum of thirty grams. The best sources are fruits, vegetables, whole grains, and especially beans. As a rule of thumb, an average serving of fruits or veggies contains about two to four grams. That means you would need the equivalent of ten servings to meet your minimum fiber requirement. Some of the best sources of fiber are corn, beans, and legumes at five to seven grams per half cup! Also, remember that it is very important to increase your water intake as you increase your fiber.

Many cultures with diets that are high in fiber (up to 50 or more grams per day) have very low rates of heart disease and cancer. Fiber is essential for good health and has been linked to the prevention of many other diseases as well. According to one study by the *Journal of the American Medical Association,* of 65,000 women ages 40 to 65, a diet high in sugar and low in fiber more than doubles a woman's risk of developing Type II (adult-onset) diabetes over a diet low in sugar and high in fiber.

So what is fiber? It is the indigestible part of plant food, and there are two kinds—soluble and insoluble. Think of the soluble fiber as a sponge that soaks up fluid and excess dietary fat as it travels through the digestive tract. Imagine the insoluble fiber like a scrub brush cleaning up the walls of your intestines as it travels the miles and miles of its journey. Fiber absorbs large quantities of water in your digestive tract. That's one of the reasons it keeps food moving through at a healthy rate.

Speaking of traveling, do you know how long it takes your food to travel from the time you eat it until its final exit? It should be about twelve to eighteen hours. That's called your transit time. A healthy transit time is important for general health and weight management.

Perhaps you can recall hearing about someone who was acutely obese and had an intestinal resection. In this operation, the surgeon ties off a segment of the intestines to decrease the absorption time of the food in the digestive tract. As a result, less calories and nutrients are absorbed. The individual must continue to eat the same volume of food to avoid becoming malnourished.

This is an extreme example of decreasing one's transit time. For good health, we don't want it to be too fast or too slow. If our transit time is sluggish, our food spends too much time in our digestive tract. Every single calorie is absorbed along with other toxins and unfavorable substances in our food.

I once heard a slow transit time compared with a big bowl of potato salad sitting in the sun on a picnic table. The potato salad builds up bacteria, has time to spoil, and loses its nutritional value. Ideally, we want a transit time that is healthy for adequate absorption of calories and other nutrients without undue exposure to the toxins in our foods, like pesticides and additives. Soluble fiber does a great job attaching to dietary fat and carrying some of it out of the body.

So how do you test your transit time? It's very, very simple . . . eat some corn and look at your watch. Now, watch for the corn and look at your watch when it arrives! That's your transit time.

Fiber is not just for regularity. It also helps notch up your energy, and that's because it slows the release of carbohydrates into your bloodstream, thus steadying your blood sugar. Let me give you an example. If you drink a glass of apple juice, the fructose (or natural fruit sugar) in the juice would quickly move into your bloodstream and your blood sugar would rise. That would give you an immediate boost of energy. But the downside is that it also falls as quickly as it rose. Within a short period of time your energy is waning. You're much better off eating an apple.

Fiber is a key to weight control. Stabilize your blood sugar throughout the day by including fiber in every meal or snack. Over time, you will be amazed at your energy level. You will probably have less sugar cravings as well. And because fiber passes through the digestive system intact, not all its calories

230

stay with the body. Fiber-rich foods typically take a longer time to eat than fatty foods, thereby providing sufficient time for satiety to be attained and overeating to be avoided. High-fiber foods also contain mass, which fills the stomach, producing a "stick to the ribs" feeling—a psychological benefit. And there are many other benefits to fiber.

- decreases fat absorption
- stabilizes blood sugar
- promotes digestion
- fills you up
- lowers blood pressure
- lowers serum cholesterol
- helps prevent digestive diseases
- promotes regularity
- contributes to bowel cleansing

—— *Quality Carbos*

Carbohydrates supply the body with its primary and preferred source of fuel—glucose. They have the most immediate and direct control on blood sugar levels throughout your day. Blood sugar (glucose) is the only source of fuel for the brain. It is stored as glycogen in the muscles and liver, and it is readily converted to glucose as blood sugar levels decrease. Carbohydrates are supplied as simple sugars in fruits, honey, sugar, and as complex carbohydrates in grains, beans, and vegetables. This mighty macronutrient also helps spare protein for use in building muscles and other protein-rich tissues.

How many carbohydrates do you need? There are varying opinions about the correct percentage of carbohydrates needed in a healthy diet. If only there were one magic formula that worked for everyone. There's not. Our needs are unique, and we all metabolize carbohydrates differently. However, fewer than

231

two hundred grams a day will cause your body to suffer something called ketosis within a few days. Ketosis occurs as a result of depleted carbohydrate stores in our body. It develops in people on fasts or very restricted carbohydrate (and therefore, high protein) diets. Without sufficient carbohydrates to support the constant need for blood sugar, brain function is compromised. It may result in lethargy, poor memory, dizziness, or other similar manifestations. The answer: Eat at least 40 percent carbohydrates daily.

For purposes of reducing heart disease, the U.S. Dietary Guidelines suggest a target of 58 percent of all daily calories from carbohydrates, preferably from fiber-rich complex carbohydrates such as fruits, vegetables, whole grains, and legumes.

My best advice as to how much you need is to experiment! Are you content after eating, or are you still searching the cupboard for something to make you feel satisfied? Only you can decide your optimum range of carbohydrates. However, a reasonable range is 45 to 60 percent of your total calories.

It's important to remember that not all carbohydrates are created equal. The proper selection can make or break your health, energy, and fat-storing capacity. Some people have become "carbohydrate sensitive" from eating too many refined products such as white bread and sugar. The body produces insulin to help deal with increasing blood-sugar levels, and it can become very efficient at converting carbohydrates to fat. Our incredibly adaptable machine is bent on survival, and survival translates to excellent fat storage. When excess carbohydrates are converted and stored as fat, 25 percent of the carbohydrates are burned in the conversion process and 75 percent are stored.

Refined grains, such as white breads, crackers, pastas, and cereals are high in complex carbohydrates—so they're just what the Food Guide Pyramid ordered, right? Not necessarily. The trouble is, unlike whole grains, refined grains have been stripped of their nutritious bran and germ. Compared to refined carbohydrates, whole grains carry loads of nutrients, and it's these "extra" nutrients that may help protect you from illness. Currently, only about one person in ten eats even one whole grain a day. The American Dietetic Association suggests three a day.

Become a bread detective! It's always a good policy to eat by color and, as a rule, brown is better. However, don't assume that beige or dark brown breads like rye and pumpernickel are whole grain. Usually the color is just dye. You need to check the ingredients. If the first ingredient doesn't include the word *whole*, the brand is using all or mostly white flour, no matter what the name implies. For example, you might find bread called "Enriched Stone Ground Wheat Bread" or "Whole Grain Oatmeal Bread," but it's not whole-grain bread if the first ingredient is enriched flour (unbleached, bromated wheat flour, stone ground, granulated, etc.). There are numerous whole-grain products on the supermarket shelves. Just read the labels before you buy.

—— *Powerful Proteins*

Protein creates a powerful nutritional base that helps stabilize blood sugar. It is also essential for tissue repair, maintenance, and growth of muscles, blood, hormones, enzymes, and antibodies. Wow, what an awesome responsibility!

When the body is low on carbohydrates or fats, protein can be broken down for energy, though it is not a preferred source. To maintain a healthy metabolism, it is important to protect your body from utilizing nondietary protein, such as your muscles, for energy.

Protein supplies four calories per gram and is the hardest nutrient to convert to fat. It takes forty calories to convert one hundred excess calories of protein into fat. That means forty calories are burned up in the conversion process! This is one reason why high-protein diets have found such popularity. Individuals can eat more calories and store less fat. However, in the long term, these diets not only become monotonous, they can also be unbalanced.

If you are eating a high percentage of protein, there is little room to include all the fiber, vitamins, and minerals you need from fruits, vegetables, and other sources. Additionally, too much protein puts an incredible workload on the body, especially the kidneys.

How much protein do you need? Protein needs may vary with the individual. You will need to experiment to see how your body best responds. We have gone from a society that ate too much protein to one of carbohydrate junkies. The best solution lies somewhere in the middle. I recommend 15 to 30 percent protein in your diet. Of course, the more physically active you are, the more protein you will need. However, some individuals do seem to respond favorably to slightly higher percentages of protein. The risk is maintaining proper balance and nutrition from a combination of all macro- and micronutrients.

The simplest calculation for ensuring that you receive an adequate level of protein is your weight divided by two. For example, if you are a woman that weighs 140 pounds, your weight (140) divided by 2 equals 70. That means you should eat at least 70 grams of protein each day.

Proteins are composed of large strings of amino acids. There are eight to ten types of amino acids that cannot be produced by the body and must be supplied in the diet. These are called "essential" proteins, and the best sources include extra-lean meats, poultry, fish, soy, low-fat milk products, and beans or legumes combined with whole grains. When shopping for meats, choose the words *loin* (tenderloin, sirloin) or *round*. These leanest cuts of beef and pork have only a little more fat than a skinless chicken breast.

The only nonanimal protein that contains all eight essential amino acids is soy. Exciting research shows that soy products provide high quality nutritional content and important health benefits for both men and women. Low in saturated fat and high in fiber, the soybean also has significant amounts of B vitamins, zinc, calcium, and iron. Soy has been proven to reduce cholesterol levels and, most importantly, is linked with a significant reduction in female-hormone-related diseases and symptoms.

In Asian countries there is no word for PMS or "hot flashes." These cultures rarely experience symptoms common to American women. One reason is because they include soy products in their daily diets. The soybean is filled with phytochemicals—some called isoflavones or phytoestrogens (plant estrogens), which seem to provide a positive sort of regulatory effect on natural hormone production. Genistein and daidzein are the most highly researched isoflavones.

In short, the potential health benefits of soy are significant. They include:

- reduced risk factors for heart disease
- reduced risk for breast cancer
- reduced risk for osteoporosis
- relief of menopausal and PMS symptoms
- may fight prostate cancer
- may protect against colon cancer
- may prevent stroke

How many isoflavones do you need? The average Asian diet includes about 100 to 130 mg of isoflavones per day. However, since soy has not been part of the American diet, experts advise consuming 60 to 80 mg per day until we know more. Also, don't overlook the fat or sodium content, which can be high in some soy products.

—— *Fabulous Fats*

Fats are fabulous for making us feel satiated and reducing our food cravings because they cause the stomach to empty more slowly. They are the most concentrated source of fuel, supplying more than twice the calories per gram of carbohydrates or protein. Except for during aerobic activity, the body prefers to store dietary fat as body fat rather than convert it to energy. Fat is essential for life. In addition to contributing to feelings of satiety and helping reduce food cravings, fat performs three primary life-supporting functions in each cell of our bodies.

1. First and foremost, fats are a ready energy source, contributing nine calories for every gram of fat used.
2. Fats act as a protective blanket shielding the organs from trauma and cold. The fat deposits surround and hold in place important organs such as the heart and kidneys. Fat below the skin helps prevent heat loss and protects against external temperature changes. (If you've ever lost a lot of weight, you probably noticed that you got cold more frequently.)
3. Fatty acids or lipids are part of every cell membrane and every organ and tissue. Fats are needed for absorption of vitamins A, D, E, and K. By assisting in vitamin D absorption, they help calcium get into the body, especially to the bones and teeth.

Research shows that people who eat smart fats like omega-3 fatty acids and monounsaturates also get less cancer, heart disease, depression, asthma, and even Alzheimer's disease. Plus, smart fats can help control diabetes and high blood pressure. Make no mistake though. Too much total fat—more than 25 percent of calories—is not good overall nutrition management.

There is no specific RDA for dietary fats, but experts recommend 15 to 25 percent of your total calories. If you are trying to lose body fat, try to keep your fat below 20 percent. Keep in mind, however, that fat can actually improve your weight management efforts because it will make you feel satiated longer. If you're struggling with feeling hungry all the time, you're probably not eating enough fat.

Eating too little fat can result in vitamin and mineral deficiencies. Many people who maintain very low-fat diets eat far too many "nonfat" foods that are high in calories. Most Americans, however, have the opposite problem—too much fat and too much saturated fat. Saturated fat can cause the most damage, raising your LDL cholesterol level (the stuff that clogs your arteries) and increasing your risk for heart disease. The average daily diet includes about 150 grams of fat, providing a whopping 1,350 calories! Still, the average person doesn't get enough of the essential fats.

Basically, our only dietary fat requirement is for the key essential fatty acids, alpha-linolenic (omega-3) and linoleic (omega-6), ranging from 2 to 5 percent of calorie intake. Deficiency of "vitamin F" (essential fatty acids) can lead to dryness or eczema of the skin, as well as to reductions in the oil-soluble vitamins A, D, E, and K. Most people need a 1.4:1 ratio of omega-3 to omega-6 fatty acids. The average American gets a 1:7 ratio.

Cholesterol

A topic of great concern in modern nutritional medicine is the correlation between increased dietary fat intake and disease—number one being atherosclerosis (clogging of the coronary arteries). These vital arteries get clogged with plaque, decreasing the flow of life-supporting blood to the tissues, which leads to high blood pressure or hypertension. This forces the heart to work harder to get blood to the body, and the constant extra effort can lead to enlargement of the heart, general heart disease, and congestive heart failure.

What is cholesterol, anyway? Cholesterol is a type of lipid or fat that performs many vital functions in your body. In fact, over 80 percent of your cholesterol is produced mostly by the liver. Only 7 percent of all the cholesterol in your body is in your blood. And when you eat less cholesterol, your body just makes more.

Cholesterol is the building block for the sex and adrenal hormones. It is the main component of bile and enables us to digest fat and fat-soluble vitamins. It coats our nerves and assists in nerve transmission. It helps the normal growth of cells and gives the skin its ability to shed water. The list goes on. The point is that cholesterol is not all bad.

But there are concerns about blood cholesterol being too high and, more importantly, having too much "bad" LDL and not enough "good" HDL. However, tests have repeatedly shown that changing your diet can only alter your cholesterol level by about 4 percent.

According to Dr. Contreras, new research indicates that it is not so much the cholesterol that is the problem, but the rest of our diets. He states that "cholesterol may be the indicator of poor lifestyle choices, but it is not the culprit itself."[4] I concur with Dr. Contreras that a total approach to healthier eating and consistent exercise will make a much bigger difference than simply tracking your cholesterol.

Eating more of the healthy fats and more whole foods full of color and phytochemicals will make a bigger impact on your cholesterol profile and your overall health. Dr. Contreras's recommendation is to cut saturated fats and increase heart-healthy fats like olive and canola oils and even butter in moderation. He states: "Let's not fall into the trap of excluding all fat from our diet. God specifically calls fatty foods like butter and curds blessings. (See Deuteronomy 32:14.) It appears that butter, long labeled an enemy of health by dieticians, is healthier than margarine."[5]

Not All Fats Are Created Equal

As you've just learned, fats are both essential to the healthy functioning of our bodies and potentially harmful, depending on the quantity and types of fat we consume. Foods typically contain mixtures of saturated and unsaturated fats and can affect your cholesterol levels differently. Remember, you want your "lows" (LDLs) to go lower and your "highs" (HDLs) to go higher.

238

Saturated fats are solid at room temperature and generally are from animal sources or tropical oils, such as fatty cuts of meat, poultry skin, whole and 2 percent milk, full-fat cheese, butter, premium ice cream, and coconut oil. Your goal should be to keep this type of fat to no more than 7 percent of your total daily calories. Here's six ways to cut saturated fats.

1. Drink fat-free or 1 percent milk.
2. Reduce cheese intake and choose reduced fat or fat free.
3. Eat meat sparingly; choose extra-lean cuts.
4. Enjoy fat-free or low-fat frozen yogurt and ice cream instead of premium brands.
5. Eat the chicken, hold the skin. You'll save half the calories.
6. Use egg whites instead of whole eggs in recipes.

Poly and monounsaturated fats are liquid at room temperature (like vegetable oils). Their properties vary. Polyunsaturated fats decrease LDL, which is good. But they also decrease the important "good" HDL cholesterol. These fats (like safflower and corn oil) are from mostly vegetable sources. Our diets today include so much vegetable oil made from corn, cottonseed, safflower seed, sunflower seed, and soybeans that we get ten to twenty times more omega-6 than the Stone Age person. Too much omega-6 hinders the work of the powerful omega-3 in your body.

Monounsaturated fats are like detergents in your bloodstream. Two excellent choices are olive and canola oils. They actually cut LDL levels without lowering HDL. They also slow the rate at which carbohydrates enter the bloodstream. Unfortunately, in America we get a third of our monounsaturates from meat, which means we also get artery-clogging saturated fat.

The American Heart Association recommends up to 15 percent of your daily calories from heart-healthy sources of monounsaturates. Some heart experts recommend even higher levels. These would include olive oil, olives, canola oil, avocados, most nuts (almonds, cashews, pecans, pistachios, peanuts), and natural, fresh-ground peanut butter.

Trans Fatty Acids

Trans fatty acids are formed when polyunsaturated oils are chemically altered through hydrogenation, a process used to turn liquid vegetable oils into margarine or shortening. A common dilemma is deciding which is better: butter or margarine. The answer is that it depends. Margarine is typically lower in saturated fat. But stick to liquid or whipped margarines whenever possible because they contain less trans fatty acids than stick margarines.

Like saturated fats, trans fatty acids tend to raise levels of LDL (bad) cholesterol and have been linked to breast cancer. Trans fats are pervasive in fried fast foods and processed foods (margarine, cookies, crackers, frozen entrees) with partially hydrogenated oil as an ingredient. Eliminate them if possible, but set a maximum intake of one gram per day.

Omega-3 Fatty Acids

To protect against fatal heart attacks, stroke, and possibly depression, breast cancer, rheumatoid arthritis pain, and severe menstrual cramps, add these powerful fats to your diet. Omega-3 fatty acids reduce the stickiness of platelets in the blood, making them less inclined to clump together and form artery-clogging plaque.

There are two sources of omega-3: seafood, which provides EPA and DHA; and plants, which have alpha-linolenic acid (ALA). If you don't eat fish two times a week, chances are you're only getting about a fifth of the omega-3 you need. Foods with high EPA and DHA are fatty fish, such as salmon and white albacore tuna, and foods high in ALA are canola oil, flaxseed, flaxseed oil, walnuts, walnut oil, and dark green, leafy vegetables. In your body, ALA is only partially converted to the more powerful EPA and DHA. Here are seven ways to get more omega-3 in your diet.

240

1. Eat fatty fish twice a week.
2. Choose salmon on the restaurant menu. A three-ounce serving will bring you almost two grams of DHA and EPA. Take home what's left for salmon burgers the next day.
3. Use canola oil for baking and cooking. Buy mayonnaise, margarine, and salad dressing made with canola oil, or try soy mayonnaise. One tablespoon of canola oil has 1.3 grams ALA.
4. Make salad dressing from walnut oil and red wine vinegar. One tablespoon of walnut oil has 1.4 grams ALA.
5. Sprinkle ground flaxseed on cereal or yogurt. Flaxseed is the plant with the highest ALA levels by far. One tablespoon has 2.2 grams.
6. Don't like fish? Take fish-oil capsules.
7. Add walnuts.

The bottom line is that your body needs some fat to function. Fat is essential for absorbing vitamins A, D, E, and K, maintaining your immune system, and keeping your skin moist. It also helps you feel satisfied longer. If you consistently eat less than 20 percent fat, you may get hungry before you have the opportunity to eat again.

—— *Vital Vitamins*

Vitamins and minerals are nutrients that are essential to health yet provide no calories. They are found naturally in foods, but the average American diet is lacking in the variety and balance of nutrients needed to keep bodies at peak performance. Supplements are an insurance policy against the reality of our busy lives.

To obtain all the vitamins and minerals necessary, an average woman weighing about 140 pounds needs approximately 2,000 calories per day of nutrient-dense foods. A man weighing about 180 pounds needs over 2,500 calories. Still, there is no guarantee of adequate vitamin and mineral intake due to less than optimal food choices, depleted soil, food processing, and other factors.

Start with the basics. Choose a multivitamin supplement that provides approximately 100 to 300 percent of the U.S. RDA for most of the following vitamins and minerals: vitamins A, E, C, D, B_1, B_2, niacin, B_6, B_{12}, folic acid, pantothenic acid, biotin, calcium, copper, iron, magnesium, selenium, and zinc.

Iron and B_6

Premenopausal women with low blood levels of iron should take a multivitamin with eighteen mg of iron. All other women need a multi with zero to nine mg of iron. Women on birth-control pills sometimes report feeling moody, grumpy, and irritable. There's a reason for this. Birth control pills lower blood levels of vitamin B_6, which helps manufacture the mood-elevating nerve chemical serotonin. Easy solution: Include B_6-rich bananas, extra lean meat, and soy in your daily diet.

It's preferable to choose a multivitamin that can be taken in divided doses throughout the day for improved absorption. Our bodies cannot absorb our total daily requirement of vitamins and minerals at one time, but it can absorb our total daily requirement in smaller doses. For example, we seem to absorb the amount of vitamin C found in an orange or the amount of calcium in a glass of milk at one time. Funny how God knew that, isn't it?

Antioxidants

Antioxidants are essential to fighting free radicals that cause premature aging and related diseases (these were discussed in detail earlier in this chapter). The most desirable source is always through quality foods. However, we cannot get all we need without including a specific antioxidant supplement in addition to a multivitamin. That's because we would need to eat the following every day to supply our bodies with enough of these nutrients:

- 1 cup sunflower seeds
- 1 cup wheat germ
- 1 banana
- 1 apple and 1 orange
- 2–3 dried apricots
- 2 T. almonds
- 1/2 cup broccoli
- 1/2 cup Brussels sprouts
- 1 cup spinach
- 1/2 cup cauliflower
- 1 medium sweet potato
- 5–6 oysters
- 1 T. blackstrap molasses
- 1 cup brown rice
- 1 cup black beans

Most of us would have difficulty eating some of these foods even once a week, let alone once a day! Antioxidant supplements include the following specific nutrients:

Vitamin A (beta carotene)	Copper
Vitamin C	Manganese
Vitamin E	Zinc
Selenium	Chromium

As with other supplements, more is not always better. Find a good quality, moderately priced supplement and take it daily. Of course, this is in addition to a diet rich in a variety of whole, live foods.

Vitamins

A substance must be essential for normal body functioning and create deficiency symptoms when removed from the diet in order to qualify as a vitamin. Vitamins work in concert with one another and other minerals, and help the body utilize food as fuel more effectively. Again, the best source of vitamins is always first and foremost—food!

Minerals

Minerals are inorganic substances that are needed in small amounts to sustain life and promote health. Like vitamins, minerals work in synergy with our foods and create a delicate balance within the body. They also work interdependently with each other and require a very specific and delicate balance. Overconsumption of one mineral easily could reduce absorption of another and result in a secondary deficiency.

There are over twenty essential minerals our body needs in small amounts, and they play a role in a variety of functions, including:

- supporting skeletal mass (calcium and phosphorus)
- being an element of blood (copper and iron)
- maintaining electrolyte balance (sodium, potassium, and calcium)
- supporting coenzyme reactions (zinc, copper, and magnesium)
- assisting with muscular contractions, nerve function, and bone formation (magnesium and calcium)

Calcium

Everyone, regardless of age or sex, needs calcium. It's the most abundant mineral in the body, making up 1.5 to 2 percent of total body weight. More than 99 percent of the body's calcium is stored in the bones and teeth. And while you know it as the

244

body's bone builder, calcium also helps your muscles contract, your blood clot, your heart beat, and your nerve impulses travel. And in kids it builds healthy teeth.

Unfortunately, 90 percent of adult women, 88 percent of teenage girls, 73 percent of adult men, and 68 percent of teenage boys are not getting enough calcium from their diets. (This is according to the USDA's Continuing Survey of Food Intake by Individuals, 1994–96.) Deficiencies may cause our bodies to rob the calcium stored in our bones, and this may lead to several short-term problems and eventually to osteoporosis. Osteoporosis literally means "porous bone," and it affects more than twenty million people in the United States. Many doctors recommend supplements for perimenopausal and postmenopausal women to help slow bone loss that comes with hormonal changes.

Your goal is to get at least 1,000 mg a day from food and supplements, and 1,500 mg for women over 50 and men over 65. Here are some quick calcium hints:

- Add nonfat, dry milk to soups, casseroles, cookie dough, and even coffee.
- Blend nonfat dry milk into skim milk to create more "whole" milk taste. Just 2 tablespoons add an extra 100 milligrams of calcium (for a total of 400 milligrams, counting the milk).
- Drink plenty of fluids to avoid constipation.
- Enhance absorption by taking your supplement with milk.
- If you take calcium and iron supplements, take them at different times for better absorption.

Iron

If you consistently experience fatigue and low concentration, the problem could be iron. This is especially true for growing children and women of childbearing age. Routine blood tests screen only for anemia, a late stage of deficiency, but you can

245

request a blood test called serum ferritin. If you are iron deficient, include more dark, leafy greens and extra lean meat in your diet. A vitamin C–rich food or drink, such as orange juice, will boost absorption of iron-rich foods.

Sodium and Potassium

These two minerals act together to form a "pump" that speeds nutrients into the cells while speeding the waste out. Congestion in the tissues will weaken this process, called the "sodium-potassium pump," and slow down the exchanges. And this is a key factor in the dreaded lumpy, bumpy cellulite formation most common in women.

Too much sodium encourages water retention and leads to decreased cell activity. Potassium naturally counterbalances sodium. The better the balance, the more efficient the "pumping" action. When this balance is disrupted by poor eating habits, excess salt in the diet, sedentary living, and other factors, sodium will draw excess fluids to the tissue spaces. This leads to congestion, slows down cellular activity, impairs the diffusion of nutrients and oxygen, and hinders cells from repairing and renewing themselves.

Zinc

Zinc is essential for growth, the repair of body cells, and energy production. It also helps your body utilize carbohydrates, protein, and fat. Zinc is found in beef, milk, cheese, yogurt, and eggs. It's less available in plant foods but can be found in whole grains. Be aware that grains lose zinc when they're processed into refined flour.

Magnesium

Magnesium is involved in more than three hundred enzymatic reactions in the body, particularly those in energy production. It's associated with growth and development, wound healing, immune system function, temperature regulation, and many activities of the brain and nervous system. Whew! The tissues with the highest concentrations of magnesium in the body are the most metabolically active—the brain, heart, liver, and kidneys. Magnesium is also essential for muscle contraction and relaxation and for production of adenosine triphosphate (ATP), the molecular energy cell needed for nearly all of the body's physical, mental, and biochemical work.

Magnesium deficiency is one of the most common nutritional challenges, particularly for the elderly. The RDA is 350 mg daily for men and 280 mg for women. The best dietary sources are tofu, legumes, seeds, nuts, whole grains, and green, leafy vegetables.

It is important to make educated supplement choices. Here are some good guidelines.

- Do not self-diagnose. Proper medical care is critical to good health. If you have persistent symptoms or illness, seek a health-care specialist before embarking on a supplement program.

- If you are currently on prescription medication, consult your doctor before making any changes. Always inform your physician of the nutritional supplements you are taking.

- Nutritional supplements work much better if they are part of a natural treatment that focuses on diet and total lifestyle.

- More is not necessarily better. Super potency, megavitamins, and therapeutic refer to doses in excess of ten times the RDA for one or more of the vitamins or minerals.

- Organic or natural are in most cases no better than synthetic. Often these terms imply a higher cost. Exceptions: chromium, selenium, and vitamin E (d-alpha tocopherol).

- Time-released vitamins and minerals in reality do not work and may even diminish adequate absorption.

- A chelated mineral is attached to another substance and can be absorbed better; however, the bond can be broken easily when the supplement hits the stomach.

- Nutrient absorption is affected more by the circumstances in which you take the supplement than by the supplement itself. Most vitamins and minerals are best absorbed with food (except iron).

- Test your vitamin's absorption. Not all vitamins break down sufficiently for absorption. One way to test your vitamin is to put one capsule in a glass of eight ounces of water and one teaspoon of vinegar. If it dissolves in twenty to thirty minutes, then your body is breaking it down and using it. If it doesn't, then request the company's disintegration tests to be sure.

Marginal deficiencies can develop over time with few clearcut symptoms. Stress, smoking, disease, air pollution, and many other factors can increase our nutritional needs over time. Good self-care requires consistent healthy living and eating.

Whew! Well, you made it through the whole chapter. And I bet you guessed . . . there's so much more I could tell you. But it's not vital right now. In fact, you may be a little overwhelmed with all this information. If so, the next couple pages will help. First, take the evaluation and see how you are doing in this area. Then, choose two to four things to work on first. Remember, you're not on a diet! You're designing a lifestyle that you can live with forever.

— Lifestyle Evaluation—Nutrition

Before you start to implement the things you have learned in this lifestyle area, begin by taking the self-evaluation on the next page. It will give you a good snapshot of your current strengths and weaknesses in this category. If you don't clearly understand your lifestyle weaknesses, it's hard to set priorities and take action.

Hopefully you took the initial evaluations in chapter 2. Now, after reading this chapter, you may see these same questions with a little more insight. Your answers will most likely be the same for now. Change will occur as you apply these principles. Take this evaluation again and every couple months to gauge your journey toward victory!

Spend about four to five minutes on the evaluation. Base your answers on your most consistent behavior or attitudes in the past three months.

Based on the last three months, please rate yourself (0–Almost never; 1–Sometimes; 2–Often; 3–Always).

_____ I think about what I eat and how it impacts my health.

_____ I have high energy to do all the things I want and need to do.

_____ I read labels and choose many foods based on that information.

_____ I eat two to three servings of fruit each day.

_____ I eat three to four servings of vegetables each day.

_____ I choose whole-grain products over more processed foods.

_____ I know how much fiber I'm eating daily.

_____ I drink ten to twelve glasses of water daily.

_____ I eat breakfast every day.

_____ I eat a good source of protein at breakfast.

_____ I choose and eat lean protein with my lunch.

_____ I limit my empty calories to less than 15 percent of my total diet.

_____ I limit caffeine and other stimulants, such as over-the-counter diet aids, especially those containing ephedra and mau huang.

_____ I take a multivitamin supplement daily.

_____ I take an antioxidant supplement daily.

_____ I choose "healthy" fats in my diet like olive or canola oil.

Add the total of all scores.

Scoring

40–48 Excellent! Your body loves you!

31–39 Good. You're on the right track.

22–30 Fair. It's time to try a little more high-octane fuel.

< 21 Poor. Your body is crying "Help!"

You've evaluated your nutrition. You've educated your mind. Now it's time to initiate a new plan. Choose from the menu of items below in the area of nutrition. What two or three things do you think would make the biggest difference in your health, energy, and waistline if you worked on them consistently? Choose those and move ahead! Transfer your top two or three priorities to the "My Nutrition Recipe" on page 252 and write one to three action items for each priority, i.e., how you're going to work these new priorities into your life.

— Nutrition Menu

—— *Wonderful Water*

Eight to twelve glasses per day
Coffee doesn't count
Carry it with you

—— *Fiber-rich*

Three to four fruits per day

250

—— *Fruits and Veggies*

Whole fruits instead of juice
Most servings one-half cup
Variety is important
Four to five veggies per day
Most servings equal one-half cup
French fries don't count
Doesn't have to be fresh

—— *Quality Carbos*

Beans and bran
White bagels and pretzels don't count
Whole grain on the label is the key
Brown rice, brown bread

—— *Powerful Proteins*

Always with breakfast and lunch
Stabilizes blood sugar
A must for muscles

—— *Fabulous Fats*

Omegas rule
Omega-6—olive and canola oil
Omega-3—fish and flaxseed
Nuts are okay—watch the cals

—— *Vital Vitamins*

Spark plugs for your body

251

Multivitamin and mineral in two doses
Antioxidants to fight free radicals
Don't overdo it. Eat good food first!

—— *Fuel and Burn*

Like a car with a five-gallon tank
Start with breakfast
Stop when you're full
Eat lighter at night

—— *Pick Your "Poisons"*

Limit junk food and chemicals
Fun food—no more than 15 percent
Artificial sweeteners—less than 3 servings a day
No sugar or caffeine until after lunch

My Nutrition Recipe

Priority   **Action**

#1_____   _____

                                           _____

#2_____   _____

                                           _____

#3_____   _____

                                           _____

#4_____   _____

                                           _____

— 13
—— you are what you
— don't eat

"Oh, my goodness, *that's* why I'm fat!" Pamela yelled so exuberantly that the whole class looked at her in awe. What great revelation had she just experienced in the middle of our lifestyle lecture? Well, she had just discovered that a few "healthy" meals she ate on a regular basis were enough calories to fuel two NFL football players for an entire game! The truth hit her like a ton of bricks. "Are you saying if I eat like this two or three times a week, I'm getting that many calories all in one sitting?" she asked me incredulously. "Looks that way," I replied. Over the next several months, Pamela trimmed down her evening meal, and her waist and hips followed. Like I've said before, it's the small stuff (and the big stuff) that you do every day that counts.

So far, we've discussed how to burn fat to the max and eat for maximum energy. Now it's time to address a few strategies for getting some unneeded calories out of your daily diet. To make this work in the long term, you need to make changes you can live with—changes that don't leave you feeling deprived or like you're on one more diet you can't wait to complete. So if eating like a naturally thin person doesn't come naturally to you, it's time to learn (and more importantly, implement) some additional techniques to balance your energy equation. I encourage you to try all these techniques and then use the ones that work best for you.

One of the most important principles I have learned in gaining control of my eating is that I always have better control when I am well rested and my energy level is high. By practicing the NutriMax Six and establishing a strong nutritional base, you'll be amazed at how many of your cravings diminish. Your increased energy will make it easier to become more active. Your activity will further increase your energy and decrease your appetite. This cycle of healthy living is one of the most effective ways to eat fewer calories. Tune in to how you feel next time you overindulge. Remember: Low energy promotes a high appetite!

— Effective Calorie Control without Dieting

—— *Daytime Eating*

Become a daytime eater. You burn calories most effectively the first twelve hours of your day. But when do you eat the most? Usually the last four hours of the day, right?

Breakfast will stimulate your metabolism and hunger early in the day. That may seem scary at first, but it will ultimately decrease your appetite later in the day. You need more calories at lunch than at dinner, so don't be afraid to fuel up for the rest of your day.

I eat a moderate-sized dinner, and only occasionally. That's because I am not very hungry after 5:00 in the evening. For me, a snack or two is sufficient most days. The "eat-burn" approach and fueling earlier in the day have helped me stay lean. How you choose to design your meals depends on your lifestyle. For some, dinner is an important family time. If this is the case for you, at least try making the meal much smaller, and whenever possible, eat it early in the evening. You'll be amazed at how one simple change can impact your body.

——— Tune In to the Hunger Scale

You learned about the hunger scale in the emotional eating chapter. If you want to get and stay lean, try to make the commitment that you will never allow yourself to feel overfull. Get tuned in to the fact that anytime you have overstuffed your stomach, you will most likely be overstuffing a few fat cells.

After years of stuffing myself until I was overfull, I began giving myself a new message that worked powerfully for me over time. It was: "I cannot stand feeling overfull. It is absolutely unbearable, so I never do it!" This may sound a bit extreme, but it has worked for me. For many years, I would repeat that phrase every time I overate. And I really feel that way now. I avoid being too full almost more than I avoid being too hungry!

However, the hunger scale alone will not ensure you have your calories under control. Some foods are so high in fat or concentrated calories that a person can eat very little and still take on too many calories.

——— Substitution

I am sure you are aware of healthier, lower calorie food choices. But you don't have to pretend to be satisfied by choosing rice cakes over tortilla chips! Frankly, as far as I'm concerned, anything that tastes like cardboard is not worth putting in your mouth.

There are many great choices available that are healthier alternatives. To me, a food must give at least 80 percent satisfaction in order to be considered "worthy." For example, there are many lower fat versions of microwave popcorn on the market. They taste great and are at least 25 percent less fat. The same goes for almost any category of packaged foods. However, despite the fact that we have more healthy food options, Americans are getting fatter. Don't overrationalize your choices. Just because something is lower in fat or calories doesn't mean you can eat unlimited quantities. In the big picture you still have to balance the energy equation.

—— *Meal Replacements*

By now, I hope it's loud and clear that I don't believe in diets or undereating. However, there are appropriate times to break some unhealthy eating cycles and make short-term eating adjustments. The use of meal replacements can break a vicious cycle. I use healthy fiber and protein shakes and high-protein energy bars for this purpose. On occasion, when I've gone a little overboard, I choose to have only protein shakes, fruit, and veggies for one to three days. It simplifies my choices and breaks the cycle.

I must stress that this is not a diet. It is a short-term attitude and intake adjustment. If you choose this technique, don't starve yourself. Just use a healthy meal replacement that simplifies your choices and breaks your cycle for twenty-four to forty-eight hours. Your cravings will be gone in no time.

It is always ideal to "eat and burn" with a balanced energy equation every day. But sometimes life is not predictable. When life gets out of balance, try meal replacements to get back in balance quickly. And remember that this is your choice. If after a couple meals you think you are in control and decide to go back to regular foods, don't feel guilty and allow yourself to get into a tug-of-war with food. These tools are meant to work for you, not against you.

—— *Portion Control*

One of the easiest ways to get a handle on the number of calories you eat without actually counting them is to practice portion control. By decreasing the amount of food you eat by 10 to 30 percent, you could save significant calories. If you had been eating an average of 2,400 calories per day, a reduction of 10 percent would result in a daily caloric savings of 240 calories. That's about 24 pounds in one year.

Consciously reduce the size of your portions whenever you serve yourself. It is always helpful to use smaller dishes, especially when you choose to indulge in fun foods. You can always have a little more later if you are still hungry. But never reduce your portions when it comes to fruits and vegetables.

Rarely is it necessary to reduce portions at breakfast either; portion control is exceptionally effective after 5:00 P.M. when we need fewer calories anyway. If all you did was cut the calories you're eating in the evening by 50 percent, I think you would find the results amazing. Try it. I'm confident it will make a huge difference in your energy equation. And if you don't get leaner practicing this technique, then it's time for the ultimate truth—count your calories!

— Calories . . . If It's Worth Eating, It's Worth Writing Down!

Accurately estimating the amount of food on your plate is a challenge. The Obesity Research Center in New York City says that people are grossly underestimating the calories they eat, by more than 50 percent in some cases.

Going back to the checkbook illustration I used earlier, just imagine living for a month without ever taking the time to subtract any of your expenditures. Guessing can be very dangerous! The best way to get a handle on what you are eating is to get a good calorie-and-food-value book and keep a journal.

I know it will feel like you are on diet for a while. But you're not. You are simply gathering information and making choices. You are validating what your body already knows—how many calories you've taken in. Why not make choices based on truth?

When I go shopping for clothes, I want to make the most of every dollar. Before I purchase a garment, I consider fashion, quality, and how much I will wear it. If I see a simple summer dress hanging in the "designer" section of the store with a five-hundred-dollar price tag, I'm probably going to look elsewhere for something comparable at a tenth of the cost. The same goes for food. Calorie awareness will help you make wiser decisions that will save you thousands of calories each week.

—— *Four Ways to Conceptualize Calories*

1. Understand what a serving is. For example, an average bagel is the equivalent of two to three servings of bread.
2. When in doubt, measure. Get an accurate picture of what a serving of your favorite cereal looks like. Learn how much space one cup of pasta looks like on your dinner plate. Pour one serving of cereal into your bowl. Is that how much you are usually eating? Probably not.
3. Read labels and interpret them accurately. Look for fat, calorie, and nutritional content.
4. Equate serving sizes with everyday items, such as:
   A deck of cards = three ounces of meat, poultry, or fish
   Your fist = one cup of rice, potatoes, pasta, or a medium piece of fruit
   Your thumb = one ounce of cheese or candy

In addition to getting a handle on serving sizes, you can begin to put foods into categories. Certain fruits or vegetables can be comparable to each other. For example, vegetables such as broccoli or cabbage can be put into one category. And I consider one cup of pasta, rice, or other grain as being in the same category. I don't have to look up every new food if I have a basic understanding of what category it best falls into.

You will have to accept that you will do a fair amount of guesstimating. Foods prepared away from home or without labels will be somewhat of a challenge. Learn to add a 10 percent padding of calories whenever you're in doubt. This will ensure that your errors will work to your advantage when it comes to slipping on your favorite jeans!

—— *A Few More Tips*

Tip #1: Read the labels of already prepared foods like lasagna, pies, frozen entrees, or other prepackaged foods. It will give you an idea of what a serving size and calorie count might be on something you make at home.

Tip #2: Use index cards to write down the calorie content of the foods you eat most frequently. Try to prepare cards for at least two or three breakfast, lunch, and dinner options. Now you have a handy reference that's easy to use.

Tip #3: Become calorie "curious" without becoming calorie "obsessive." If it's too hard to figure out calories at a given snack or meal, just do portion control. Calorie counting does not have to be an all-or-nothing venture.

Tip #4: Challenge yourself to count calories for one month as if it were a business project that will produce a great bonus at the end. (And it will. The bonus will be a loss of fat and gained insights into how to keep it off.)

If I didn't convince you earlier of the importance of a reality check, let me reemphasize that now. This short-term exercise will have a profound effect on your choices for the rest of your life. Determine to take this short educational course in "calorie physics." Write down everything you eat and compute your calorie intake. Take on the attitude that if it's worth eating, it's worth writing down. You can look up and compute your calories as you go or you can calculate them at the end of the day.

The key to effective portion control and calorie counting is complete honesty. It is very easy to rationalize your own version of truth. Just keep reminding yourself that truth is not relative. Your body knows it; your fat cells reveal it! Being honest with yourself may seem like an enormous task at first. However, I guarantee that you will more clearly understand the role your choices are playing in changing on your body. In no time, you will have a very clear concept of what you are really eating and burning. I have seen this exercise have a dramatic impact on the attitude and choices of many people.

Note: For many years, I have used my Caltrac Activity Monitor to give me an accurate assessment of my daily calorie burn. It also allows me to input my calories as I eat. It tells me if I am ahead of the game or behind by giving me the net excess or deficit of calories all day long. I've found this very helpful, and so have many of my clients.

— Planning for Success

Your success in developing a healthy approach to cutting calories depends on your willingness to change your old ways of doing things. And the best way to avoid eating disaster is to be prepared! The following ideas will ensure you are prepared for anything.

——— *Meal Planning*

It will take a little time for you to develop a lifestyle of eating that is both satisfying and effective in helping you burn off excess fat. But there is no single plan that will work for everyone. You must plan your eating based on your likes, dislikes, lifestyle, and objectives. Each time you decide to have a meal or snack, you must decide what choices will best meet all your objectives. Consider these factors:

- What sounds good?
- How hungry am I?
- How many calories have I burned?

260

- How many calories will I burn?
- How many calories can I afford to eat?
- What do I feel like?
- Is there adequate protein and fiber to stabilize my blood sugar?

Where's the meal plan? Did you notice? I haven't included any specific eating plans, menus, or recipes. What's the deal? How are you going to eat?

Well, you are going to design your own plan. Why? Because my purpose is to educate you so that you can make food choices that will work for you. Make your choices based on the health you want, the body you want, and the lifestyle you want. It's highly unlikely that you will eat based on prepared meal plans for the rest of your life. To lose weight permanently, you need to get it off the same way you plan to keep it off. And no one can tell you how to eat for life . . . except you. At a point, you'll need to figure out what works for you, what calorie-cutting methods you choose to use, and what foods you feel are worth the investment. As far as I'm concerned, that time is now.

My objective is to give you strategies to help you design that plan, and the following ideas may be helpful. You don't have to write out detailed eating plans to lose excess fat. Make the best choices you can moment to moment and move more every day!

Breakfast

As you learned in the NutriMax Six, breakfast is the meal that jump-starts your metabolism for the day. It's important to fuel up within the first two hours of waking even if you don't feel hungry. Try to include protein and fiber with each meal. Avoid simple sugars and caffeine early in the day to ensure a stable blood sugar.

Lunch

Lunch should be your most substantial meal. It needs to sustain you through your busy day, and it will impact your hunger in those dangerous hours in the evening. Lunch is an excellent time to include a little more protein—lean poultry and fish or lots of beans and legumes. Planning will ensure that you make healthy choices. Include leftovers from previous dinners or choices from healthy restaurants.

Snack Options

Remember it's best to fuel and burn with frequent, small meals all day long for maximum energy. And it's good to have healthy snack options with you. I like good energy bars with adequate protein and a little fat (there are some good chocolate-covered options on the market). They satisfy my hunger and sweet cravings, and the protein stabilizes my blood sugar. It's also a good idea to bring along a sturdy piece of fruit, like an orange or apple, for a quick snack when you're on the go. Nuts are also a healthy, satisfying, easy-to-carry snack. Just be careful you don't go nuts with the nuts—the calories add up fast!

Dinner Options

Dinner traditionally has been our main meal, but if you think about it, there is no need to fuel up for rest, relaxation, or sleep. This meal should be taken as early in the evening as possible and kept fairly light. Consider it roughly one-fifth of your daily calories or a maximum of about four hundred to five hundred calories on an active day. If you like an evening snack, make dinner even lighter.

—— *Dining Strategically*

Dining out doesn't need to feel like you've lost control. By understanding nutrition basics, you can eat almost anywhere healthfully. Don't be afraid to ask for what you want; you are the customer. Here are ten ways to dine strategically.

1. Decide beforehand what kind of food choices you will make.
2. Be assertive in requesting your food servings and preparation.
3. Consider sharing or ordering half portions.
4. Ask how much fat is used in preparation and, if necessary, ask for it to be reduced.
5. Have the waiter remove your plate as soon as you feel full.
6. Never go out when you're a 1 on the hunger scale.
7. Avoid the words *fried, breaded, creamed, au gratin,* and *a la mode!*
8. Remember that white sauces are always richer than red.
9. Ask for your salad tossed with a half portion of salad dressing or pasta with half the sauce.
10. Ask for nutritional information; most restaurants have it available upon request.

—— *Surviving Special Occasions*

Holidays and special occasions almost always include special (high calorie) food. Whenever you attend a party or special event, there are several strategies that can help you take control of your calorie intake. First, never starve yourself beforehand. That is a sure way to increase the chance of a blowout! Here are seven ways to survive special occasions:

1. Start the day with a great breakfast and practice the Nutri-Max Six.
2. Offer to bring a low-calorie snack or contribution to the meal.
3. Brush your teeth just before the event. Food just doesn't taste as good after brushing.

4. Don't stand near all the goodies.
5. Spend more time talking than eating.
6. Drink plenty of water or club soda to keep you hydrated and full.
7. Don't hesitate to leave food on your plate.

—— *Condiments and Concentrated Calories*

There are some foods we need to put on what I call the "condiment list," such as cheese, olives, bacon, and other high-calorie foods. Flavor your foods with these rich treats, but try not to make them a substantial part of your meal or snack. Also be careful to eat things like avocados and nuts with care. They are healthy, but they also are concentrated calories.

It goes without saying that other high-calorie fun foods like candy, cookies, and pastries add up fast. There are no forbidden foods, yet these rich and satisfying treats can make a big dent in your calorie bank account. I encourage you to get tuned in to how much fat and calories are really in that mud pie and chocolate cheesecake they serve at your favorite restaurant. The truth will scare you into sharing your dessert and even leaving a few bites on the plate!

—— *Shopping for Success*

To keep your calories under control, you must have a wide variety of excellent choices at hand. Plan a day when you can spend an extra thirty or forty minutes in the grocery store "exploring." You will be amazed at some of the new foods that are great alternatives to some of your old (more fattening) favorites. Shop with a mission and make sure you never enter a grocery store hungry. Here are six additional shopping strategies.

1. Plan your meals and snacks.
2. Make a list.

3. Shop with focus.
4. Avoid danger zones.
5. Never shop with kids!
6. Say no to impulse buying.

—— *Practice Calorie Busting*

There are unlimited ways to reduce calories and fat from your food. From buttering your toast to preparing a gourmet meal, you can use creative techniques to make delicious and healthier alternatives. In fact, I have observed that if many people simply start "spreading" lighter, they'd be lighter also! Take a look at how much peanut butter, mayonnaise, or jelly you put on your bread. How much dip is on that healthy veggie? "Go light . . . get light" is a great motto.

— Taking Control of Calories

Here are ten tips I've learned that will help you take control of your calories.

1. Build an "appetite control foundation" by eating and sleeping for maximum energy.
2. Avoid going to a 1 or 5 on the hunger scale.
3. Have healthy and enjoyable snacks with you at all times to avoid crisis eating.
4. Become more of a daytime eater. Try decreasing your evening intake by 25 to 50 percent.
5. Practice portion control. (Not with breakfast or plant foods . . . but everything else!)
6. Substitute lower calorie and fat choices whenever possible.
7. Use replacements to break a bad cycle for twenty-four to forty-eight hours.

8. Plan for calorie success by developing a strategy for special occasions.
9. Count calories for at least a month to get the truth.
10. Balance your energy equation for maximum energy and minimal body fat.

You can find many excellent light-cooking magazines or cookbooks at any local bookstore. They are full of healthy, calorie-busting ideas. I've included fifty-two of my favorite suggestions for you here.

1. Eat your toast with jam and no butter or margarine.
2. Poach (don't fry) your eggs. Cut whole-grain, unbuttered toast into squares and put your eggs on top. Or scramble one yolk and two egg whites in a nonstick pan.
3. Snack on thirty-five pretzel sticks instead of one ounce of potato chips.
4. Hard candy or mints are low in calories and satisfy the sweet tooth. They also take about three to four minutes to eat.
5. Graham crackers with warm herbal tea satisfy sweet cravings with less sugar and fat.
6. Try dried fruit instead of candy or cookies.
7. Lender's bagels are smaller and less calories than most. Use jam or low-fat cream cheese and spread lightly.
8. You can easily save hundreds of calories weekly by reducing the amount of butter, mayonnaise, and other spreads on your breads, rolls, etc. The spread should blend into the surface of your food. Scrape off any excess with your knife before you take the first bite.
9. Choose rolls instead of high-fat biscuits.
10. Leave the cheese off your sandwich and add tomatoes, cucumbers, or pickles.

11. Learn how to read your labels correctly for fat and calorie content. If a food is more than 30 percent fat, don't buy it.
12. Love cheese? Select parmesan or low-fat mozzarella. Buy sharper cheeses for more flavor, and use less.
13. Never eat regular mayonnaise. Cut low-fat mayo with Dijon mustard to decrease the calories and increase the flavor. There are also many other flavorful, lower calorie spreads on the market. Try a new one each month.
14. Cranberries on chicken or turkey sandwiches are good year-round. Plenty of moisture, so your sandwich needs very little mayo!
15. Carry your own reduced-fat salad dressings. There are too many tasty and healthy dressings now available to ever settle for high-fat choices.
16. Reduce the frequency of red meat in your diet and eat smaller portions. (Six ounces is plenty at any one time.)
17. Angel food cake can be dressed up in many ways for a low-fat dessert. Try making a chocolate angel food—yum!
18. Choose lower fat cookies such as biscotti, vanilla-filled wafers, Oreos, and meringues.
19. Low-fat frozen yogurt with special sauce or flavor is a wonderful treat. Try fruit sorbet with berries.
20. Avoid the guacamole and stick with low-calorie salsa. If you can't resist the avocado, mix it with generous amounts of salsa and fresh tomatoes.
21. Whenever possible, use cheese and nuts as condiments. Cut the amount in recipes in half and limit snacking on these high-fat morsels to one ounce at a time.
22. High-fat chips and buttery crackers can pile on the calories quickly. If you can't eat just three or four, avoid them. Or try to measure out an ounce into a ziploc bag for strategic portion control when you're on the run.
23. Artichokes with low-fat mayo or low-calorie dips are nutritious and delicious.

24. Jicama cut in sticks adds flavor and variety to vegetable plates.
25. Substitute ground turkey for beef. Brown and rinse with hot water in a colander to remove excess fat. Save about 160 calories per pound!
26. Use low-fat or nonfat options whenever possible in recipes.
27. Orville Redenbacher Smart Pop is a great-tasting, reduced-fat popcorn.
28. Thicken cream sauces with 1 percent milk and cornstarch instead of butter and flour.
29. There is no reason to eat high-fat ice cream—ever! There are too many excellent low-fat and nonfat alternatives.
30. Croissants contain about three hundred calories from fat. They're not worth it! Stick with your favorite fresh bread.
31. Order pizza with thin crust, one-third less cheese, and lots of veggies. Save about 100 to 150 calories per slice.
32. Can't resist your occasional potato chip? Try the baked options and save both calories and fat.
33. Use less low-fat mayonnaise in tuna or chicken salad by adding a little fat-free rice vinegar.
34. Never butter your pancakes, waffles, or French toast. Just top with reduced-sugar syrup or jam. Pancakes are generally the lowest calorie choice. Make your own in a nonstick pan.
35. Always select red sauce versus white with your pasta. White sauce = cream = fat!
36. Reduce the amount of meat or poultry in your fajitas, casseroles, or other dishes and increase the vegetables, rice, or beans.
37. Choose eggplant or vegetable lasagna instead of regular.
38. Try frozen grapes for a fun snack.
39. Try Land O' Lakes light whipped butter. Only thirty-five calories per tablespoon!

40. All tortillas are not equal. Read the labels and buy the smaller, low-fat selections. Buy beans without added fat or lard. Remember, cheese is a condiment.
41. Eat a turkey sandwich instead of chicken salad. (Save two hundred to three hundred calories.) In fact, never order tuna or chicken salad when you are dining out. Most restaurants use full-fat mayo, and lots of it!
42. At your favorite fast-food restaurant, choose the smallest burger, light on the sauce, and hold the cheese. When they ask, "Want to super size?" the answer is "Never!"
43. Have you had your eighty ounces of water today? It's free!
44. Choose tuna packed in water instead of oil.
45. Order a regular taco instead of super. Hold the sour cream, please!
46. Add an extra two cups of beans to your turkey or chicken chili.
47. Extra hungry tonight? Have a large sweet potato or yam with your chicken breast or entree.
48. Bake a big, fluffy potato and stuff it with low-fat cottage cheese, chives, and top with a little sharp cheddar. Very satisfying.
49. Choose BBQ chicken instead of pork or beef.
50. Always remove the skin off chicken before eating.
51. Fresh herbs and feta cheese flavor up pasta without all the oils.
52. Eggnog-flavored coffee creamer is a lot less calories than eggnog. Make a fresh cup of coffee with special flavor for dessert.

— 14
—— use it or lose it . . .
— lifestyle fitness

Do you get winded climbing a single flight of stairs or have difficulty keeping up with your husband on a brisk walk around the block? Have you ever felt like you are going to collapse from exhaustion after spending the day sightseeing? If your fitness level is so low that you have to go into training simply to go "power shopping," you need to read this chapter now!

On the other hand, perhaps you've been committed to a regular exercise regime for some time. But your body still isn't changing. You're in the gym three times a week, and you know you're healthier because of your commitment, but your body still looks the same. Read on . . . you may find some answers to your dilemma.

God designed our bodies to respond to consistent stimuli in a purposeful way. When you participate in regular weight-bearing exercises like walking, they stimulate your body to build stronger bones. Why? Because the regular "pavement pounding" tells your body to get ready for more, and it prepares you by giving you more of what you need—stronger bones and bigger muscles. Pretty cool, huh? That's why I've titled this chapter "Use It or Lose It"—use the muscles, bones, cardiovascular system, and lungs God gave you by developing an active, vibrant lifestyle. This in turn will energize and mobilize your body to become all it was designed to be. Or otherwise sink into an increasingly sedentary lifestyle and watch your body transform into a living, breathing marshmallow.

In the journey to fine-tune your fitness to your desired level, you can apply some basic principles that will help you toward your goal. Our bodies were designed for consistent activity. Just as we need food and water every day, we also need activity to stimulate muscle and bone growth and to keep our metabolisms running efficiently.

Lifestyle fitness is about getting in tune with your body and making some decisions about what you want and need it to do for you. Decide to make exercise a part of your life forever. You wouldn't forget to eat or brush your teeth, would you? Think of your fitness in the same way!

As I have said before, your body is your vehicle for life. Do you want to live in a fine-tuned, high-energy sports car or a broken down jalopy? I'm sure you want a body full of energy, one that burns lots of calories and feels strong and fit. The good news is that you don't have to become an elite athlete or exercise fanatic to feel that way.

My friend Melody began her lifestyle journey about a year ago. She wanted to lose weight and get healthier so she would be around to watch her beautiful little granddaughters grow up and get married some day. This is what she shared with me recently:

"I'd reached a point in my mid-fifties where I was feeling decidedly 'old.' I'd had a hysterectomy, and an old back injury was starting to talk to me a bit more loudly than it used to. I didn't like how old I was feeling, but I tried to convince myself it was normal. But it just didn't feel that way. One day I was playing with my granddaughters and realized that if someone yelled,

'Gramma! Go long!' I couldn't do it. I couldn't even follow them around the zoo for the afternoon any longer. "A year later and thirty-five pounds lighter, I'm a new person. I discovered that it does matter what you eat and how much you exercise. Little things do make a big difference. I began to exercise daily, eat less fat, drink more water, and eat more whole foods. Today, I feel ten years younger than the last time we went to the zoo. In fact, my (younger) husband has trouble keeping up with me! I realized that I do have control over things like aging and that I can make myself much more productive and energized. It's not about losing weight any longer; it's about maximizing my energy, giving myself endurance and flexibility that I haven't had for years. And using my body feels absolutely terrific!"

— Benefits of Exercise

Many people report feeling less stress, irritation, depression, and anxiety following regular exercise. And there is also an extra benefit of improved self-esteem, mood, and an enhanced ability to concentrate. These benefits result in part from endorphins, which are chemicals in the body that give you a "high" feeling after exercise. They also help relieve body aches and pains.

This chapter will help you understand the key components of fitness. It's been my experience that trying to learn specific exercises from the pages of a book is very difficult. So my objective is to give you a clear understanding of how your body works and what you need to be fit for life.

There are a multitude of exercise programs available in illustrated books and video programs, and at local gyms and health clubs. Explore your local resources to find a program that meets your personal and financial needs. Exercise professionals, such as certified trainers, group class instructors, or even professional videos can demonstrate proper form and help you make corrections in your technique when you are getting started.

273

Toward the end of this chapter I will give you my unique, effective, and very time-efficient workout. But don't skip ahead! I have some important teaching to do first.

—— *Get Moving*

Lifestyle fitness is not difficult or complicated. Simply by getting more active, you are taking a positive step toward a lifetime of healthy and fit living, and understanding the physiology of how your body best burns stored fat will motivate you to move more. For those of us who love food and want to be lean without dieting, the truth is this simple: We must become more active and purposely move most days for the rest of our lives!

Now don't let that scare you. You don't have to become a fitness fanatic. But increasing your daily activity and calorie burn is essential. You may notice that I do not always use the word *exercise*. This is because some of you may not be comfortable with that word. I do believe in the value and long-term benefit of exercise. However, I do know people who have lean, healthy bodies and never break a sweat.

In some cases, certain individuals have learned the benefit of "cumulative activity." This means that their activities of daily living are so consistently active that they use all their major muscle groups and burn significant activity calories every day. But unfortunately, active living does not always come easily. The nature of our jobs, schedules, and other factors has reduced our activity level to almost nothing.

If leading an active, calorie-burning existence is a challenge for you, or if *exercise* is a negative word, your self-talk may be sabotaging your success. It is important to start changing the messages you are telling yourself. Comments like "I hate this, but I know it's good for me" or "I can't wait until this workout is over" are not going to reinforce new habits.

What is your excuse? Write down three reasons why you find it difficult to keep fitness a priority in your life.

1.

2.

3.

Now rewrite those three excuses to become a positive statement or affirmation. For example, "Exercise bores me" could be rewritten to say, "I enjoy exercise and the way it makes me feel." It may seem odd telling yourself a "lie." But it will become real to you when you change your mind by filling it with healthier messages. And wouldn't it be great to enjoy exercise?

Now it's your turn. Rewrite those three messages below.

1.

2.

3.

By replacing old, negative messages with new, positive ones, you will start building excellent neuron pathways to your success. Imagine yourself enjoying how your body feels and the new strength and endurance you've achieved. Every time you get up and get moving, imagine all those stored fat cells just waiting in line, ready to jump into your bloodstream and get metabolized for energy!

—— *Keeping Yourself on Track*

I've come up with several ways to keep yourself on track and focused on your goals.

- Establish realistic goals.
- Use a log to track your progress.

- Reward yourself when you accomplish a goal.
- Tailor your program to your needs, lifestyle, and physical ability.
- Be flexible and realistic.
- Fight boredom with diversions like music and television.
- Develop a network of workout partners.

Before starting an exercise program, it's wise to get a medical checkup in order to avoid aggravating any existing conditions such as heart disease, high blood pressure, or back problems. If you're over forty or have an ongoing physical condition or other limitation, definitely see your physician before starting an exercise program.

— Total Fitness

There are three components of overall fitness: (1) strength and toning, (2) aerobic endurance, and (3) flexibility.

By understanding the role each component plays, you can design your own active lifestyle and become a calorie-burning machine. Whether you choose to join a gym, get a personal trainer, or just engage in fun activities on a regular basis, you will have the knowledge to fine-tune your fitness to meet your personal goals.

—— #1—Strength and Toning

Muscles are your body's engine. They are metabolically active, and they not only burn calories during physical activity but also when your body is at rest. Increasing your muscle mass will increase your body's capacity to burn calories. One pound of fat only burns about three calories per day. But one pound of muscle burns up to fifty calories! If you gain two pounds of muscle over the next year and nothing else changes, you could lose about ten pounds of body fat.

Some studies show that exercise can increase your resting metabolic rate by up to 20 percent. In addition, fat-releasing enzymes are manufactured in muscle cells. The more fit and toned your muscles are, the more effective they are at releasing those fat-releasing enzymes.

It has been proven that diets, which significantly restrict your caloric intake, can cause the loss of lean muscle mass. Strength training helps maintain your lean muscle mass while you lose fat, and it is excellent for toning and shaping the body and preventing injuries. It also helps the following conditions:

- osteoporosis
- arthritis
- obesity
- aging
- hypertension
- high cholesterol

To build strength, a muscle must be overloaded or worked beyond its normal level. This overloading challenges your muscles on a regular basis and stimulates them to build stronger and tighter muscle fibers. This is best accomplished through some form of resistance training, in which you can use free weights, machines, exercise bands, or even your own body weight.

You do not have to join a gym. There are many simple exercises you can do in your own home using inexpensive equipment and your own body weight for resistance. The first time I ever entered a gym to lift weights, I was able to bench press my own body weight. I didn't know it at the time, but this was excellent. My fiancé (now husband) was completely blown away and asked me when I had started lifting weights. I hadn't been lifting weights, but I had been doing push-ups for over five years and "pushing my weight." I had no idea how strong I had become. Strength training does not necessarily mean you will build large muscles (women, by nature of their hormones, rarely do this). First your flabby, untrained muscles will get tighter and take up less space. Then, depending on your sex, body type, level of resistance, and frequency of workouts, you may begin to see an increase in size. But you are in control of your results. Muscle tissue begins to atrophy within forty-eight to seventy-two hours. If you feel too bulky, just reduce the frequency and intensity of your workouts— your muscles will begin to shrink without consistent stimulation. But they will never turn to fat. And fat cannot turn into muscle, no matter how hard we work out. Fat is fat and muscle is muscle!

If your body still has a fat layer over the muscle, you will not see the benefits of all your work initially. However, beneath the surface, important things are happening. Your increased metabolism and fat-releasing enzymes are increasing the "melt rate" of fat from your body. You will be seeing some of those toned and fit muscles showing under your skin before you know it.

Before you pick up one weight or start getting to work on your trouble spots, it's important to understand that there is no such thing as "spot reducing." When evaluating your body, you are most likely unhappy with the fat that is lying on top of the muscle, and you may feel compelled to do lots of leg exercises or sit-ups. Those exercises are fine for the muscles, but no matter how many times you kick or crunch, the fat is just going for a ride. If you want to see toned muscles, you have to lose the excess fat that is lying on top.

—— *#2—Aerobic Endurance*

Fat burns best during aerobic activity. The word *aerobic* means to use oxygen. Large-muscle, sustained activities are considered aerobic because we can sustain them for long periods of time without running out of oxygen. When the activity is iso-

278

lated to a single muscle group, as in weight lifting, or when we exercise so hard we become winded, this is considered anaerobic, or without oxygen.

Aerobic endurance is a measure of how fit your heart and lungs are. Aerobic exercise causes you to breathe more rapidly and your heart to pump more quickly. With regularity, your body will respond with lower body fat, heart rate, cholesterol level, and blood pressure. Another positive benefit is increased energy and endurance.

To improve cardiovascular fitness, you must engage in sustained aerobic activity for at least twenty minutes, three times per week. This is the bare minimum. Most people need to move more than that to maintain a lean body.

Aerobic exercise elevates your metabolism while you are exercising and keeps it elevated for some time afterward. The level of after burn is dependent on the duration and intensity of the exercise. Aerobic exercise also stimulates other systems in your body that burn calories. The result? You become leaner!

The percentage of fat burned for energy steadily increases from about 5 percent fat and 95 percent carbohydrates to over 50 percent fat and 50 percent carbohydrates in the first thirty minutes of aerobic activity. This fifty/fifty ratio continues from the thirty-minute point throughout the aerobic workout. It's easy to see that the most efficient and healthy way to access stored body fat is through frequent aerobic exercise.

Certain types of aerobic activity are more effective than others for weight control. You should pursue those activities that put the least amount of stress on your body. You may have heard these referred to as "low impact" or "nonimpact."

Examples of low-impact aerobic activities:

- walking
- step aerobics
- low-impact aerobic dance

Examples of nonimpact aerobic activities:

- swimming
- bicycling
- rowing

Since one goal of aerobic exercise is to strengthen the heart, it must be challenged sufficiently to stimulate change. Monitoring your target heart rate is one of the safest and easiest ways to ensure cardiovascular fitness. Your objective is to work between 60 and 75 percent of your maximum heart rate.

If you are just beginning a fitness regime, start slow at a 60 percent target heart rate. As your fitness increases, you can work toward a higher level. Count your pulse by placing two fingers (not your thumb) over your radial artery inside your wrist or at the carotid artery at the side of your neck, under your chin. Never check your carotid artery by pressing on both sides of your neck at once. Your brain does like an ample supply of oxygen at all times, and that could slow the flow a bit!

Calculating Your Target Heart Rate

220 minus your age in years = your maximum heart rate
Maximum heart rate x .60 = your target heart rate, low range
Maximum heart rate x .75 = your target heart rate, high range

Example:

220 – 35 = 185   Target heart-rate range
185 x .60 = 111
185 x .75 = 139   111 to 139

Another easy way to monitor your level of aerobic activity is called the "Perceived Exertion Scale." The scale is rated from 1 to 10. Consider an exertion level of 1 as if you were asleep and 10 as if you were running for your life!

Perceived Exertion Scale

1. Sleeping or comatose
2. Barely moving
3. Very weak
4. Weak
5. Moderate
6. Somewhat strong
7. Strong
8. Very strong
9. Very, very strong
10. Maximum—run for your life!

People who exercise regularly between 4 and 7 on this scale can significantly lower their risk of cancer and heart disease. Fitness levels that improve longevity can be reached easily by most men and women who simply walk briskly for a total of thirty minutes or more four times each week. These benefits can also be realized by breaking exercise into two or more sessions, such as three ten-minute segments. As you add aerobic activity to your lifestyle, monitor your exertion during the activity to make sure you are exercising safely.

—— *#3—Flexibility*

Muscular flexibility improves your posture, appearance, and overall performance. By staying flexible, you can decrease the risk of joint injuries and muscle strains. When you have engaged in too much activity, stretching can also help reduce muscle soreness. As you get older, your flexibility naturally decreases. However, with a regular stretching program, you can slow down the process and stay quite flexible. Females generally have more flexibility than men.

It is important to stretch properly to avoid injury. Ballistic (or bouncing) stretching is not recommended; static stretching that holds the muscle in one position without bouncing is best. And stretching is more effective when you warm up properly first. Warm muscles will relax and lengthen much more readily.

Cross-training refers to a training technique that periodically varies the type and intensity of your exercise. There are several advantages to cross-training. First, the variety allows you to use a wider range of muscle groups, which enhances overall fitness. Secondly, cross-training helps prevent overuse injuries that are a result of doing the same thing over and over. Lastly, and perhaps most importantly, cross-training stimulates your metabolism.

Our bodies are incredibly adaptable machines. If we keep doing exactly the same thing (such as walking or running each day), over time our bodies will burn approximately 25 percent less calories while doing that activity. For those of us who are trying to burn maximum calories, this is not good news!

The best way to ensure that your body remains a Ferrari is to mix up your aerobic workouts now and then. If you mostly walk, try swimming or biking once or twice a week. If you prefer aerobic classes, try a rowing machine or Nordic Track occasionally.

— Danna's TV Workout

After more than twenty years of teaching group aerobic classes at a variety of athletic clubs and gyms, I was ready to do my own thing. The music and group energy had served its purpose to keep me motivated for years. Being the instructor was certainly a great motivator to get me to class without excuses! However, we all need to realize that there are seasons to our workout regimes.

A few years ago, I decided I needed a more time-efficient exercise plan. I realized that by the time I packed up my gym bag, jumped into the car, and drove back and forth to the gym, I could have a decent workout done. So a few years ago, I started to work out at home more often than not. And my most important piece of exercise equipment became my television remote control! That is, I do 90 percent of my exercise while channel surfing all the early morning news and talk shows. They are a great distraction from my workout and keep me informed as to what's going on in the world.

—— *The Warm-Up*

Even when you are doing your own thing, it's still very important to start with a warm-up. I begin by moving around the house, going up and down my stairs; making the bed; whatever gets my circulation pumping. If I'm ready to just jump in right after jumping out of bed, then I warm up by walking in place until I feel my muscles loosening up. If any muscle group (especially my legs) feels tight, I do specific stretches for those areas.

—— *The Aerobic Phase*

With remote in hand, I'm ready to burn some calories. Ideally, I like to burn four hundred to five hundred calories before I jump into the shower. I've used a Caltrac Activity Monitor for years to tell me exactly how many calories I burn, but if you don't have a monitor, you can simply use a clock and decide how long you want to work out aerobically. I recommend a minimum of fifteen minutes. Once you've built up your endurance, thirty or more minutes will help you maximize the fat-burning benefit of your workout as I taught you in chapter 11.

I use a variety of movements during my aerobic phase. Depending upon your fitness level, you can walk or jog in place, step side to side, alternate high-knee lifts, or perform any other type of aerobic move you've learned. Be careful not to be too repetitive, especially when first starting out. It is very important to vary your movement to avoid overuse injuries. Pay special attention to the tightness of your muscles the next day and stretch accordingly.

You can also use a portable step to add variety and another low-impact option. If you are exercising on a hard surface, it is important to use only low-impact moves. This means you should always have one foot on the ground and avoid a lot of bouncy moves. Highly padded carpeting can also be a problem. While it may seem like the extra cushion is good, you can still suffer injuries because of the lack of stability and how your body lands on that type of surface. Shoes are just as important in this type of workout as they are for a jog around the block, so put them on and replace them regularly.

—— *Tone and Stretch*

It is also fun to do light conditioning exercises using hand weights while watching your favorite program. Imagine if you committed to doing at least five minutes of sit-ups and a few leg exercises every time you watched television in the evening. Wow! It's so easy and effective. Your clothes would fit better in no time, and you wouldn't feel guilty for being a couch potato.

Once or twice a week, I encourage you to have an extra-long stretch session in front of the TV. Start at your neck and work your way to your feet, stretching every muscle group along the way. You will feel both relaxed and invigorated in the process. And it is a great way to prevent injury and diminish stress.

For me, combining television with my workout makes the time fly, and I don't feel guilty wasting time just vegging in front of the tube. Even when I'm exhausted at the end of a hard day, I sometimes forgo the aerobic workout and simply stretch or do some light floor exercises while I watch a favorite program. Another positive variation is to combine your exercise time with "catch up" time with family members. The key is to find enjoyable, time-efficient ways to work fitness into your lifestyle.

— An Ounce of Prevention

There is nothing more frustrating than getting injured once you begin to enjoy the benefits of your fitness investment. Start slow and listen to your body. The old motto "No pain, no gain" is a fallacy.

Follow the guidelines noted in this section to protect yourself from injury. Include a warm-up, cool-down, and stretch segment in every workout. Additional stretching and a day off should be included any time you feel significant muscle tightness.

Cardiac alert! The greatest risk of cardiac arrest is not during intense exercise but at its conclusion. Your body must make major adjustments as your heart rate slows and circulation changes. Always take at least three to five minutes to walk slowly or march in place at the end of an aerobic workout. Check with your physician if you notice any shortness of breath, chest pain, or pressure. Don't ignore your body's messages! It is better to be safe than sorry.

Shoes. Shoes are an important investment. Make sure they fit properly and are designed for your particular activities. Shoes often need to be replaced before they look worn, because they begin to lose their support and shock-absorbing qualities long before they lose their tread. If you can, invest in two pairs and rotate them.

"RICE" for injuries. Rest, ice, compress (wrap), and elevate any injury to minimize its severity. For best results, immediately elevate the area, use ice to decrease inflammation for the first twenty-four hours, and seek medical attention if it is more than a simple strain. Don't keep exercising! Endorphins pumping into your system during exercise may mask the pain, so don't get a false sense of security. Stop your workout and give your body twenty-four hours to tell you if it's okay.

Breathe. Our need for oxygen increases dramatically with exertion, so remember to breathe, fully expanding your abdomen and exhaling completely. You should be able to engage in sim-

285

ple conversation during your activity. If you become breathless or light-headed, slow down and pace yourself. If you're getting a side ache during activity, you are not breathing properly or you are working too hard.

Practice "belly breathing." Inhale through your nose and focus on letting your abdomen expand as your lungs fill. Holding in the abdomen and filling the chest limits the amount of oxygen you can take in. So fill up fully and give your body plenty of air.

Stand up. Posture is also important at all times and especially during your workout. Your torso should be erect, shoulders back and head up. Concentrate on keeping your abdominal muscles pulled in firmly to support your lower back. (Just be sure to let them expand as you breathe!)

Good posture immediately improves your appearance and sense of well-being. You won't get fatigued as quickly or be as prone to backaches. And, of course, strong abdominal muscles are essential to good posture and a healthy back. So don't neglect your sit-ups!

— Getting Started Safely

Making the decision to start exercising is the first step, but consistency is the key to realizing measurable benefits. You don't need to overdo it! It is better to get a light, twenty-minute workout three or four times a week for the rest of your life than to work out intensely every day for a month. Remember that this is a lifetime venture.

Make sure you are not hungry before your workout. A light snack thirty minutes beforehand will provide you with sufficient energy for the activity. Your fat-burning efficiency is actually improved if your body is well fueled.

Warm up and stretch your muscles daily to increase flexibility and elasticity. Exercise does not have to be painful in order to be effective. You should notice an increased alertness and energy after exercise. If you don't, you may have worked too hard, too long, or without enough fuel.

Get your lifestyle into the act as well. Here are some simple ideas on how to do this.

- Use the stairs instead of the elevator.
- Get rid of the TV remote control—unless you are exercising in front of the TV!
- Park at the back of the parking lot.
- Take a walk on your lunch break.
- Take walking visits with your friends.
- Have walking meetings whenever possible.
- Pace when you have to wait for someone.
- Do gardening or yard work.
- Clean up the garage. (At least you'll burn calories!)
- Play ball with the kids or the dog.
- Take active outings like trips to the zoo.
- The list goes on and on!

It's also very important to develop healthy attitudes and habits. Here are some ways to do this.

- Decide to make exercise a permanent part of your life.
- Identify and work on any self-talk "speed bumps."
- Set manageable and realistic goals.
- Make an appointment with yourself daily.
- Select activities that you enjoy.
- Incorporate strength, endurance, and flexibility into your routine.
- Try cross-training to maximize benefits and minimize injury.
- Do at least one thing—move aerobically.

- Start out slowly!
- Listen to your body.
- Make it enjoyable so you will keep doing it day after day.
- Realize that any exercise is better than no exercise at all.
- Find and use fitness resources.

Sometimes we need to take small steps toward strengthened and toned muscles. Here are some ways to do this.

- Take a toning class or buy a good exercise video.
- Consider a personal trainer for two or three sessions.
- Start with weights and repetitions that are comfortable for you. You can also learn simple exercises using your body as weight.
- Put abdominal strength at the top of your list. Learn and do safe sit-ups at least three times a week. Strong abdominal muscles will support your lower back and improve your posture. When you stand tall with your stomach pulled in, you look ten pounds leaner!

It's also important to take some small steps toward aerobic endurance.

- Start with as little as fifteen minutes of low-intensity aerobic activity, three times a week. Gradually progress to a minimum of thirty minutes of moderately intense aerobic activity five or more times a week. Remember that fat metabolism maximizes to about 50 percent after thirty minutes of aerobic activity.
- Start each aerobic segment at a comfortable pace, allowing your cardiovascular system to adjust and your muscles to warm up fully. If you feel stiff or sore, slow your pace down and allow your heart rate and breathing to adjust to the activity.

- Keep moving steadily for at least the first three minutes. Once the muscles are warm, they will stretch much more effectively. If you feel any area of tightness, stop and stretch, holding each position for fifteen to thirty seconds.

Walking is one of the easiest ways to begin your aerobic training. Almost everyone can do it. There is very little risk of injury, and it is easy to pace yourself. Walking is low impact and requires little or no stretching, unless your muscles feel tight. It burns as many calories as running when you cover the same distance. For example, you burn the same number of calories walking a mile as you do running a mile. You just get there faster when you run! In fact, walking at a fast pace is a more difficult workout than a slow run.

For cardiovascular fitness, walk four days per week. For weight loss, try to walk every day to keep your metabolism stimulated and your activity calories high. If you're a beginner, start with one mile or less and gradually increase your distance. Walking is convenient because you can do it anywhere. Wear a supportive, flexible shoe and enjoy the sights!

Here are some small steps you can take toward a flexible and injury-free body.

- Incorporate a full body stretch into your fitness routine three or more times each week.
- Stretch after a two to five minute, low-intensity aerobic warm-up and again after your cool down.
- Stretch slowly without bouncing.
- Hold each stretch for fifteen to thirty seconds and then gradually release back to the starting position.
- Pay special attention to hip, lower back, hamstring, and quadriceps muscle groups.
- Tune in to your muscles. They will tell you what they need.

289

To achieve total fitness you need a combination of strength, aerobic endurance, and flexibility activities woven into your lifestyle. With consistency, you will start to notice changes in how your body looks and feels. Each day you will feel stronger and more energetic. Consistency is the word you need to remember; every day counts.

Hopefully you took the initial evaluations in chapter 2. Now, after reading this chapter, you may see these same questions with a little more insight. Your answers will most likely be the same for now. Change will occur as you apply these principles. Take this evaluation again and every couple months to gauge your journey toward victory!

— Lifestyle Evaluation—Fitness

Based on the last three months, please rate yourself (0–Almost never; 1–Sometimes; 2–Often; 3–Always).

_____ I crave activity and find ways to move more each day.

_____ I enjoy exercise and how it makes my body feel.

_____ I have high energy to do all the things I want and need to do.

_____ I make exercise and activity a priority in my life.

_____ I understand the need for aerobic, strength, and flexibility training.

_____ I engage in aerobic activity four or more times per week.

_____ I take the stairs or park far away whenever I can.

_____ I monitor my heart rate and know I am exercising safely.

_____ I am injury free and able to engage in most activities.

_____ Being healthy and fit is important to me.

_____ I listen to my body and know what it needs.

_____ I wear appropriate and quality shoes for exercise.

_____ I have a very active life and am moving throughout the day.

_____ I work out my major muscle groups two to three times each week.

_____ I can easily touch my toes without bending my knees.

_____ I maintain strong abdominal muscles.

_____ Add the total of all scores.

Scoring

40–48 Excellent! You're a fit machine!

31–39 Good. Stay consistent.

22–30 Fair. Use it or lose it!

< 21 Poor. Take one small step and start moving!

— Fitness Menu

—— *Aerobic Fitness*

Level 1: Fifteen to twenty minutes three times per week

Level 2: Twenty to thirty minutes five times per week

Level 3: Thirty or more minutes six to seven times per week

—— *Strength and Toning*

Level 1: Abdominal workouts every other day

Level 2: Abdominal plus leg toning every other day

Level 3: Abs and legs every other day; upper body toning alternate days

—— *Flexibility*

Level 1: "Warm" and stretch tight muscles before workouts
Level 2: Stretch before and after every workout
Level 3: Three or more stretch and posture sessions per week

—— *The Lifestyle*

All activity counts. So move, move, move!
Never sit if you can stand.
Never stand when you can walk.

—— *Advanced Fitness*

Cross-training to enhance overall fitness
Interval training for variety and strength
Specific sport-training and strengthening
Distance running or competitive training

—— *Aches, Pains, and Limitations*

Take care of problems first.
Prevention is essential—broken bodies slow you down.
Seek the advice of professionals and follow that advice.

My Fitness Recipe

Priority   **Action**

#1 _____   _____
                          _____
                          _____

#2 _____   _____
                          _____
                          _____

292

#3_____   _____
                              _____
                              _____
                              _____

#4_____   _____
                              _____
                              _____
                              _____

Some Ways to Burn 100 Calories*

Activity	Duration	Cals Burned
Biking	15 min.	96
In-line skating	15 min.	104
Jogging (moderate)	10 min.	100
Jumping rope (moderate)	10 min.	100
Walking (12-min. mile)	15 min.	113

Estimates based on a 130-pound female. The more you weigh, the more you'll burn.

— 15
⸺ words for the walk

— Victory at Last!

The restaurant was one of the best in San Diego. The menu was expansive with so many wonderful choices. But that wasn't why I couldn't seem to make a decision. It had been hours since lunch, but for some reason I wasn't particularly hungry. Nothing appealed to me at that very moment. I ordered an appetizer and salad just to be polite and marveled at the new woman who said no to a five-course meal simply "because."

Now, don't get me wrong. I still love food. It's just that I don't love it all the time. I'm easily satisfied and content. My body and mind seem to sing in concert at just the right time, "Enough is enough." I can't tell you how liberating it is to be at this point. Twenty years ago, the thought of staying lean for decades and, more importantly, feeling released from the bondage of my food obsession seemed impossible. I'm here to tell you that it is not.

However, this journey is not simply about changing your mind using some sort of mental manipulation. Remember that melodic, catchy tune from the '80s, "Don't Worry, Be Happy"? The song made it seem like the key to happiness is simply a decision. I'm thinking the guy who sang the song was happy not so much from his attitude but more likely from what he was smoking. Have you ever noticed how long that kind of "happiness" lasts? A little child vacillates quickly between happy and sad. Food, toy, comfort—happy. No food, broken toy, wet diaper—sad. And it doesn't change much as we get older; we just raise the satisfaction bar a few notches. Nice car, chocolate, beautiful home—happy. Car broken down, on a diet, small apartment—sad. And even the "good" stuff doesn't satisfy for long. The more we have, the more we want. The bigger, nicer, richer, the better. That's human nature.

—— *I Want . . .*

Do you doubt me? Make a list of all the things you plan to buy in the next month. Now, next to each item mark an "N" for need or a "W" for want. It's a need if it supplies your basic requirements for food, shelter, or clothing. Everything else is a want. Sure, some things are more important than others. But how many things on your list could you live reasonably well without? I looked at my list and saw that I didn't even need all the food items written down. But I did want those peanut butter cookies. They would make me very happy . . . for a few minutes.

As Americans, we've been hearing all our lives about how we have the unalienable right to "life, liberty, and the pursuit of happiness." Yet those of us who have lived long enough realize that life is unpredictable and often painful. Happiness is illusive, and mountaintop experiences are few and far between. As we mature, most of us know that fulfilling our short-term want lists has left us . . . wanting.

We must realize that losing weight and keeping it off will not make us happy. Deep, abiding joy is found in something much more lasting. As I've said before, the journey toward a victorious lifestyle is about changing from the inside out. You will take quite a few detours along the way, and some days will be easier than others. But every little victory adds on to the next.

Ultimate victory is not about this or that program working for you. Programs don't work; people do. And people plugged into the mighty power of an almighty God can be transformed beyond their wildest imaginations when they allow themselves to be conformed to his image rather than the image of the world.

Isn't that what will really bring us lasting victory? When we seek God first with our hearts, souls, minds, and strength? And he is faithful to meet us right where we are.

We've covered a lot of ground on this journey. From healthy thinking to burning fat, from eating healthy to getting fit for life, I've given you dozens of principles and strategies to fight the battle of the bulge. But, more importantly, I hope you have discovered (or perhaps rediscovered) the most important principle of all . . . seeking the "one thing" first. Intimacy with God is the ultimate goal. It is the only thing that will satisfy.

— The Joy Factor

Focusing on a deep, abiding relationship with Christ is so satisfying that it leads to something much greater than happiness. When we focus on Christ, we find what the Bible calls "joy." Happiness is a positive emotional response to positive circumstances, but joy is a deep, abiding satisfaction *despite* our circumstances. Since so much in life is out of our control, it makes sense to seek joy.

As you continue on this lifetime journey toward a healthier you, inside and out, I want to remind you of the most life-changing principle of all. Make it your life's passion to become God-obsessed. Try to practice the presence of God each and every day by

- praying as if it is the air you breathe;
- worshiping the Lord and experiencing the refreshing living water that he alone can provide;
- nourishing your mind and spirit with God's Word; and
- digesting its truths through quiet meditation until it transforms your life.

In times of quiet mediation, God draws near to us as we draw near to him. In these times, he has helped me to put this crazy life into perspective. He has helped me see my struggles with better clarity. He has helped me accept that which I cannot change and depend upon him for that which I can.

I once wrote a poem that came in those quiet moments. The poem is simply the words of a surrendered heart realizing it has no ultimate control. And that is a very safe place to be.

Molded by the Master

Here I am, a lump of clay,
what would you have me be today?
Form me, mold me, make me whole,
I trust you with my life, my soul.
Teach me just which ways are yours,
to walk through only godly doors.
Wisdom, peace, and joy abound
when I walk your solid ground.

Spirit of the living God,
Holy Lord who shed his blood;
Purify my heart with fire,
that I may seek what you desire.

Black and white, I take a stand,
grayness abolished by your hand.
Trusting in your promised word,
I walk by faith with hope assured.

At last, I know your plans for me.
It's not to be a mystery.
To love, to serve, and trust each hour,
guided by your awesome power.

                                    Danna Demetre

— Do You Know Him?

You picked up this book and realized pretty quickly that I
truly believe there is very little meaningful change that can be
accomplished apart from God. Sure, you can go through all sorts
of exercises in self-discipline and personal motivation. But if
you've read even part of this book, you've seen that I believe all
external change leaves us only temporarily satisfied. I'm not saying that we shouldn't care about our health and appearance. It's
just secondary to things that will never pass away—our souls
and spirits.

So I cannot close this book without sharing the truth that sur-
passes everything else: God loves you and wants to have a relationship with you—a personal, intimate, life-changing relationship. If you are not positive that you know God intimately
through the sacrifice of his Son, Jesus Christ, then I challenge
you to ask yourself what you believe. If you were to die today
and God were to ask you, "Why should I let you into heaven?"
what would you say?

The familiar verse John 3:16 tells us how to receive eternal life.
"For God so loved the world, that He gave His only begotten Son,
that whoever believes in Him shall not perish, but have eternal
life." It's that simple. Believe in the Son. Later in John 14:6 Jesus
says, "I am the way, and the truth, and the life; no one comes to
the Father but through Me." God never refuses to save anyone
who believes. Yet he does not force anyone to accept him either.

Once we truly understand that God's holiness and our imper-
fections are incompatible, we begin to appreciate why Christ

came and died. In Romans 3:23, the Bible says, "All have sinned and fall short of the glory of God." That means everyone. And the most common sin of all is self-sufficiency. We don't think we need God. The Bible also says in Romans 6:23 that "the wages of sin is death." (That is, eternal separation from God, a.k.a., hell.)

The rules governing who goes to heaven and who goes to hell are established by God's nature and are unchangeable. He is the judge and jury. A perfect sacrifice for sin is required, and that sacrifice is Christ. If you accept his death as the payment for your sin—past, present, and future—you are cleansed and made holy.

Christ not only died but rose from the dead to new life. When you believe, you experience a spiritual birth and are reborn as a child of God; hence the term "born-again Christian." In John 3:3, Jesus said, "Truly, truly, I say to you, unless one is born again he cannot see the kingdom of God." Through faith in Christ, you experience a fundamental change in your nature so that you can now coexist with a holy God.

You don't have to pray a formal prayer, walk down an aisle, or perform a ritual. You don't have to be in church. You can be driving in your car, working at the office, or sitting in the comfort of your home. You don't have to clean up your act first, either. Believe me, you can never be good enough! God doesn't require you to *do* anything. Just recognize and believe in your heart that the work has already been done through the sacrifice of Christ. When you have heard the truth, it is time to make a decision. The apostle Paul writes in 2 Corinthians 6:2 that God has said, "At the acceptable time I listened to you, and on the day of salvation I helped you. Behold, now is 'the acceptable time,' behold, now is 'the day of salvation.'"

None of us know when our time will be up, but we do know that day will come. Heaven is most simply defined as where God is. It is a place of rest, glory, purity, fellowship, and joy in the presence of God. Hell is a place of eternal separation from God and all that is good. It is a place reserved for people who have been judged and found guilty of unbelief—those who die without trusting Christ as Savior.

Christ's desire to rescue you from hell motivated him to die an excruciating death for you. The precise moment you place your faith and trust in the work and person of Jesus Christ is when you are born again and begin an intimate relationship with God through Christ—for all eternity!

notes

Chapter 3: *The Battle of the Body*

1. Oswald Chambers, *My Utmost for His Highest* (Grand Rapids: Discovery House Publishers, 1963), 131.
2. Ibid.

Chapter 4: *Sweat the Small Stuff*

1. The Caltrac™ Activity Monitor is manufactured by Muscle Dynamics Fitness Network in Torrance, California.
2. Charles R. Swindoll, *Strengthening Your Grip* (Nashville: W Publishing Group, 1982), 206–7. Used by permission.
3. Francisco Contreras, M.D., *The Hope of Living Long and Well* (Lake Mary, Fla.: Siloam Press/Strang Communications Company, 2000), 93.

Chapter 5: *Balancing Body, Soul, and Spirit*

1. Edwin Louis Cole, *Profiles in Courageous Manhood* (Tulsa: Albury, 1998), 25.
2. Stephen R. Covey, *The 7 Habits of Highly Effective People* (New York: Simon & Schuster, Inc., 1989), 146.
3. Bruce Bickel and Stan Jantz, *God Is in the Small Stuff* (Uhrichsville, Ohio: Promise Press, 1998), 97.

Chapter 6: *Discovering Your True Identity*

1. Viktor E. Frankl, *Man's Search for Meaning* (New York: Washington Square Press, Simon & Schuster), 1963.
2. J. I. Packer, *Knowing God* (Downers Grove, Ill.: InterVarsity Press, 1973), 37.

3. Timothy R. Scott, Ph.D, "Come Home," *Purpose 5*, no. 3 (2002): 7–9. Dr. Scott holds a Ph.D. in New Testament Theology and is senior pastor of Scott Memorial Community Church in San Diego, California. He is also president of Declare His Presence Ministries in San Diego and host of *Dr. Scott Live!* a daily Christian radio talk show on KPRZ 1210 AM, Salem Communications. Web site: www.DeclareHisPresence.org.

4. William Backus, *The Healing Power of the Christian Mind* (Minneapolis: Bethany, 1996), 133.

5. Timothy R. Scott, personal interview, 2002.

Chapter 7: *Building a Healthy Body Image*

1. Diana Twadell, "Beautiful People," *Purpose* 3 (San Diego: Women of Purpose, summer 2000), 4, 10.

Chapter 8: *You Are What You Think*

1. Bob George, *Classic Christianity* (Eugene, Ore: Harvest House, 1989), 9.

2. Backus, *The Healing Power of a Christian Mind*, 9–10.

3. Ibid., 14.

4. Ibid., 72.

Chapter 9: *The Battle of the Flesh*

1. George, *Classic Christianity*, paraphrased from 137–38.

Chapter 10: *Overcoming Emotional Eating*

1. Charles Stanley, televised sermon, 20–26 September 1998.

Chapter 11: *Burning Fat to the Max*

1. Patti Tviet Milligan, R.D., M.S., is the nutritional consultant for LifeStyle Dimensions. She has more than twenty years experience, specializing in nutritional science and preventative medicine.

Chapter 12: *You Are What You Eat*

1. James F. Balch, M.D., *The Super Antioxidants* (New York: M. Evans and Company, Inc., 1998), 6.

2. Francisco Contreras, M.D., *A Healthy Heart* (Lake Mary, Fla.: Siloam Press, 2001), 102.

3. Balch, *The Super Antioxidants*, 16.

4. Contreras, *A Healthy Heart*, 69.

5. Ibid.

Danna Demetre is the Christian woman's total life coach. She has a great passion for encouraging women toward greater balance of body, soul, and spirit through her writing, speaking, and radio ministries. She has combined her professional knowledge with her personal experience to become a healthy role model for women of all ages.

Danna is president of Lifestyle Dimensions, a company dedicated to helping others make healthy and lasting lifestyle changes. She is also president and cofounder of Women of Purpose, an evangelistic outreach ministry committed to encouraging women toward life-changing freedom in Christ. In addition to a busy speaking ministry, Danna produces a daily Christian radio talk show and is the host of a weekly health show called *Healthy Solutions*.

Danna and her husband, Lew, have three grown children and a six-year-old adopted grandson, Jesse. They live in San Diego, California. Danna can be reached at www.dannademetre.com or by e-mail at dannademetre@cox.net.